SECOND EDITION

Documentation Manual For
Writing SOAP Notes
in Occupational Therapy

SECOND EDITION

Documentation Manual For
Writing SOAP Notes
in Occupational Therapy

Sherry Borcherding, MA, OTR/L
University of Missouri
Columbia, MO

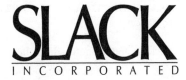

An innovative information, education, and management company
6900 Grove Road • Thorofare, NJ 08086

ISBN-10: 1-55642-719-0

ISBN-13: 9781556427190

Printed in the United States

Published by: SLACK Incorporated
6900 Grove Road
Thorofare, NJ 08086-9447 USA
Telephone: 856-848-1000
Fax: 856-853-5991
www.slackbooks.com

Borcherding, Sherry.
  Documentation manual for writing SOAP notes in occupational therapy / Sherry Borcherding. -- 2nd ed.
    p. ; cm.
  Includes bibliographical references and index.
  ISBN 1-55642-719-0 (alk. paper)
  1. Occupational therapy--Documentation--Handbooks, manuals, etc. 2. Medical protocols--Handbooks, manuals, etc. 3. Medical records--Handbooks, manuals, etc.   I. Title.
  [DNLM: 1. Medical Records--Handbooks. 2. Occupational Therapy--methods--Handbooks. 3. Patient Care Planning--Handbooks. 4. Writing--Handbooks.   WB 39 B726d 2005]
RM735.4.B67 2005
615.8'515'068--dc22
                              2005009933

Last digit is print number: 10 9 8 7 6 5 4 3 2 1

DEDICATION

This book is dedicated to Jan, who carries on the family tradition in Occupational Therapy.

Contents

ACKNOWLEDGMENTS

Many people have contributed to the development of this manual. First, I would like to thank Diana Baldwin, Director of Occupational Therapy at University of Missouri, for her patience in teaching me how to teach. Without her nurturing and support, I might have taken another pathway entirely. Thanks to Fred Dittrich for moving me as gracefully and quickly into the Information Age as I could tolerate. Thanks to Sandy Matsuda for her editing contributions, and for her loving friendship and support. Thanks to Doris O'Hara for bequeathing me the basic course material many years ago, and to Charlet Quay, Stephanie Owings, David Lackey, Lynne White, LeaAnn Brittain, and Carol Kappel for filling in the gaps in my knowledge base. Thanks to Leanna Garrison for being the Format Goddess. Thanks to Theresa Lackey, Chris Nelson, Linda Eagle, and Randy Kilgrore for their help and support. But most of all, I would like to thank the occupational therapy classes at the University of Missouri–Columbia who allowed their notes to be used to teach others.

ACKNOWLEDGMENTS

ABOUT THE AUTHOR

Sherry Borcherding currently serves as a faculty member at University of Missouri–Columbia, a Carnegie Research Extensive University, where she has taught since 1992. She teaches disability awareness, complementary therapy, and a three-semester fieldwork sequence designed to develop critical thinking, clinical reasoning, and documentation skills. She has also taught clinical ethics, frames of reference, psychopathology, loss and disability, long-term care, and wellness. Two of her courses are designated as campus writing courses and one is credentialed for computer and information proficiency. Sherry is frequently invited to present on collaborative learning, peer review, and educational technology.

Sherry graduated with honors from Texas Woman's University with a BS in occupational therapy and went on to complete her master's in special education with special faculty commendation at George Peabody College in Nashville, TN. Following her staff positions in rehabilitation, home health, and pediatrics, she assumed a number of management roles including Chief Occupational Therapist at East Texas Treatment Center, Director of Occupational Therapy at Mid-Missouri Mental Health Center, and Director of Rehabilitation Services at Transitional Housing Agency. She has also planned, designed, and directed occupational therapy programs at Capital Regional Medical Center in Jefferson City, MO and at Charter Behavioral Health Center in Columbia, MO.

Besides teaching, Sherry consults on quality assurance issues for local behavioral health centers and has a private practice devoted to complementary and alternative therapies. She is certified in CranioSacral Therapy at the techniques level through Upledger Institute and is attuned as a Reiki master. For leisure, Sherry enjoys folk dance, music, and all kinds of three-dimensional art. Her pottery has appeared in several local shows over the past few years.

Chapter 1
Documenting the Occupational Therapy Process

Introduction

Welcome to a new style of writing. The first time you see an experienced occupational therapist make an entry in a health record, you might be tempted to think you will never be able to do it. Just the technical language alone can be intimidating, and then there is the amazing attention to detail in the client observation, the insightful assessment, and the plan that just seems to roll off the therapist's pen while you are wondering how long it will take you to be able to predict a course of treatment like that.

Professional documentation is a skill, and like any skill, it can be learned. Learning a skill, whether it is downhill skiing, playing the violin, or composing a progress note requires two things of you: instruction and practice. This manual is designed to get you started with both parts of the process. Information is provided on each part of the documentation process, and the worksheets are designed to let you practice each step as you learn it.

SOAP Notes

Although occupational therapists write in more than one format, this manual presents a systematic approach to one form of documentation, the SOAP note. The manual is designed as a teaching tool and is most effective if used as a workbook, reading the information in each section, completing each exercise, then checking your answers against the suggested answers in the Appendix. The material presented here grew out of a course on documentation taught to seniors at the University of Missouri–Columbia, a Carnegie Research Extensive University. It has been field-tested to be sure it is understandable and effective in helping you learn both documentation and clinical reasoning skills.

SOAP is an acronym for the four parts of an entry into the health record. The letters stand for Subjective, Objective, Assessment, and Plan. These terms and their origins are further explained in the next chapter. The format for writing SOAP notes taught in this manual is one that is reimbursable under both Medicare Part B and managed care. While all notes written in occupational therapy practice settings do not have to meet these requirements, the Medicare Part B and managed care standards are the most rigorous. If you learn to meet these standards, you are not likely to be denied reimbursement by any third party payer. Current occupational therapy practice is in many ways determined by which services are reimbursable, and documentation of client care is the vehicle by which that service is communicated. Many therapists were never taught how to write effective notes and had to learn it on the job. They have learned what works in their own situation, but may or may not be prepared to meet the requirements of other settings.

Our Evolving Professional Language

The World Health Organization (WHO) has developed a common language for thinking about the outcomes of our services (Mandich, Miller, & Law, 2002). *The International Classification of Functioning, Disability and Health* (ICF) provides a systematic classification system for anything that a human being can do, as well as any possible disturbance of these functions (WHO, 2001). Functional states are divided into three dimensions:

1. Body functions and structure
2. Individual activity
3. Participation in society

These three may be influenced by **environmental** factors. All body, activity, and participation dimensions have two poles, one end indicating a limitation, and the other end indicating positive or nonproblematic factors. The WHO model tells us that health is influenced by more than body structures; it is also impacted by the ability to participate in roles and carry out desired activities. Intervention may be aimed at the impairment level (client factors), the activity level, or the level of social participation (WHO, 2001).

"The evolution of our professional language" has been described by Youngstrom (2002b, p. 607) as reflecting the changes in what occupational therapists do, and in how we describe it. In 2002, the American Occupational Therapy Association (AOTA) adopted *Occupational Therapy Framework: Domain and Process* (Framework) (AOTA, 2002a). This document, which is frequently called the *Framework*, describes the domain of occupational therapy as "engagement in occupation to support participation in context or contexts" (AOTA, 2002a, p. 610). It also describes the process that constitutes best practice in occupational therapy. The *Framework* brings the language that occupational therapists and occupational therapy assistants use in documentation into alliance with WHO concepts (Delany & Squires, 2004). Occupational therapists are no longer content to see health as the absence of impairment. We now are returning to our roots, and to a view of health that is based on a broader definition—a definition that includes interaction with the environment and satisfaction with overall quality of life.

The *Occupational Therapy Practice Framework*

The *Framework* provides a multilevel model for understanding the domain of occupational therapy (Youngstrom, 2002b). In this model, the occupations of the client are primary. The ability to engage in occupation rests on the client's **performance skills** in the areas of motor, process, and communication, as well as on the **performance patterns** of habits, routines, and roles. The performance skills and patterns in turn rest on **context, activity demands,** and **client factors** (Figure 1-1).

By doing an **occupational profile,** we are able to determine whether any contextual features, activity demands, or individual client factors need to be addressed, depending on the occupational needs of the client. The occupational profile is a client-centered approach to gathering data (occupational history, experiences, interests, habits, and patterns of daily living), as well as what the client needs, values, or hopes to gain from the present situation, allowing the client to set priorities for treatment. Throughout the intervention process, the occupational profile is refined and the targeted outcomes are updated in accordance with changes in the client's condition and changing priorities (AOTA, 2002a).

Clients engage in meaningful occupation in a variety of arenas, or **contexts.** For example, a context may be physical (such as home or office), social (such as family or colleague), or virtual (such as the Internet). If a client is being seen in a context such as a hospital or clinic that is not usual for him, it is important to determine whether or not the skills you are teaching are transferable. A client who has good functional mobility in the hospital may be completely stopped by three steps into a mobile home or a 24-inch door into the bathroom.

Client factors refer to the client's anatomy and physiology, and include such things as sensation, range of motion (ROM), and amputation. If these do not limit the client's ability to self-select his or her occupational tasks, they do not necessarily need to be assessed or addressed in treatment.

Activity demands are interactive and are most easily thought of in terms of task analysis. The demands of an activity include both what is needed to perform the activity, and how that relates to the client's stated goals.

Engagement in Occupation to Support Participation in Context or Contexts

Performance in Areas of Occupation
Activities of Daily Living (ADL)*
Instrumental Activities of Daily Living (IADL)
Education
Work
Play
Leisure
Social Participation

Performance Skills   **Performance Patterns**
Motor Skills   Habits
Process Skills   Routines
Communication/Interaction Skills   Roles

Context   **Activity Demands**   **Client Factors**
Cultural   Objects Used and Their Properties   Body Functions
Physical   Space Demands   Body Structures
Social   Social Demands
Personal   Sequencing and Timing
Spiritual   Required Actions
Temporal   Required Body Functions
Virtual   Required Body Structures

* Also referred to as basic activities of daily living (BADL) or personal activities of daily living (PADL)

Figure 1-1. Domain of occupational therapy. Reprinted with permission from American Occupational Therapy Association.

The content of this manual reflects the scope of occupational therapy practice and emphasizes the basis of our services as described in the *Framework* (AOTA, 2002). It also incorporates concepts and guidelines found in:
- *The Reference Manual of the Official Documents of the American Occupational Therapy Association* (AOTA, 2004b)
- *The Guide to Occupational Therapy Practice* (Moyers, 1999)
- *International Classification of Functioning, Disability and Health* (ICF) (WHO, 2001)

The standards for educational programs in occupational therapy specify that the student will "document occupational therapy services to ensure accountability of service provision and to meet standards for reimbursement of services. Documentation shall effectively communicate the need and rationale for occupational therapy services" (Accreditation Council for Occupational Therapy Education [ACOTE], 1999, Section B.4.10). This manual will provide you with a tool for becoming competent in these skills.

Engaging in Meaningful Occupation

Before we talk about documenting the occupational therapy process, we need to differentiate occupational therapy from other disciplines in the health professions. Occupational therapists and occupational therapy assistants provide interventions for people who have problems engaging in an **area of occupation**. This is important to note, because this is what we will document. When documenting occupational therapy services, the focus on ability to engage in occupation is critical for showing the necessity for occupational therapy and for preventing any question of duplication of services (Youngstrom, 2002b). Those entities and agencies that provide reimbursement for occupational therapy services have differing priorities, and it is crucial to know your payment source when documenting your services (Lloyd, 2004; Thomas, 2003). Each payer has an interest in different areas of occupation, and will reimburse services that are aligned with those interests. The *Framework* describes seven areas of occupation.

Activities of Daily Living

Basic or personal activities of daily living (ADLs) are necessary tasks for self-care and personal independence. These are tasks such as bathing, grooming, hygiene, dressing, eating, toileting, communication, sleep, sexual activity, and functional mobility. It is important to consider not just the physical ability to care for self, but also other components, such as cognition, that might cause limitations in performance. For example, rather than being unable to perform grooming skills due to a physical factor, a client might fail to notice that his poor hygiene is problematic. If your services are being reimbursed by Medicare, you will often find yourself writing goals for ADL activities.

Instrumental Activities of Daily Living

Instrumental activities of daily living (IADLs) require more complex problem-solving and social skills, including such tasks as money management, cleaning, laundry, child care, driving, shopping, and meal preparation. Therapists who work with persons with brain injuries also talk about executive functions that are at issue in frontal lobe damage. Executive functions involve planning, goal setting, and organizational tasks, which impact ability to perform IADL tasks effectively. If your client population has cognitive involvement, you may find that your goals include many IADL activities.

Work

Work includes seeking and carrying out paid employment, as well as participating in volunteer experiences. Work is a primary area of occupation for adults and forms a part of adult identity. If your services are being reimbursed by worker's compensation, you will find that your goals and interventions center around return to work. If vocational rehabilitation is your payer, you might find instead that your work goals involve helping prepare a client for work that is both meaningful and within his or her capabilities.

Leisure

Leisure activities are those intrinsically rewarding things we do when we are not obligated to be doing anything else. Particularly for older people, leisure is a very important area of occupation. Leisure and play, especially for adults, are generally considered activities that enhance one's quality of life, and are not regarded as being reimbursable goals. However, the performance skills and patterns required for leisure activities are transferable to a variety of occupations that are reimbursable. For this reason, leisure is usually approached indirectly in documentation, with a focus on performance skills and patterns.

Play

In a young child, play may consist of organized tasks such as games with rules or spontaneous activities such as exploratory play. One of the primary occupations for a child is acquiring those skills necessary to progress through age-appropriate developmental milestones, and these skills are acquired through play. If you are working with young children, you will often find yourself talking about play in your documentation.

Education

Education is another of the primary occupations of a child. Those activities and skills needed to perform successfully in formal or informal educational settings are unique. Services to children in the educational system are for the purpose of the child performing school-related activities. If you are working in school-based practice, your goals and interventions must relate to skills and behaviors needed in the classroom to be reimbursable.

Social Participation

As social beings, people need to be able to interact successfully with others and to keep their behavior within the contextual norms of the community, the family, and peer groups. If you are working with clients who have developmental disability, brain injury, or mental health problems, you might find yourself documenting goals and interventions for social participation.

Skilled Occupational Therapy

Throughout this manual, occupational therapy service is described as **skilled occupational therapy**. This term originated in Medicare regulations that define the difference between skilled and nonskilled services. Since Medicare Part B requirements are being followed in this manual to insure that your services will not be denied payment, it is important to know that Medicare reimburses those interventions that are identified as skilled and does **not** reimburse those considered nonskilled. **Skilled** services are those that require decision making and highly complex competencies and that have a well-defined knowledge base of human functioning and occupational performance. **Nonskilled** services are defined as those that are routine or maintenance types of therapy, both of which could be carried out by nonprofessional personnel or caregivers. The use of "skilled" in this manual emphasizes the necessity of documenting your occupational therapy interventions clearly as those activities requiring the services of a qualified occupational therapist or occupational therapy assistant (Lopes, 2000). In long-term care settings, Medicare is becoming more stringent in determining where the skill of an occupational therapist is no longer needed. For example, you may be reimbursed for only one visit for exercise or two to three treatment sessions for positioning. In this situation, you are expected to develop the intervention or prevention program, with follow-up provided by nonskilled personnel. It is necessary for you to document in a way that differentiates your skill as an occupational therapist from that of nursing or restorative services. Your documentation should demonstrate the level of complexity or sophistication of the services you are providing.

Other Reimbursable Services

Safety Concerns

The ability to perform a task must include the ability to do it safely. Safety concerns such as a high probability of falling; lack of environmental awareness; severe pain; the lack of skin sensation; abnormal, aggressive, or destructive behaviors; or suicide risk all fall within the scope of skilled occupational therapy. Intervention strategies targeting safety are usually seen by third party payers as a cost-effective service because they prevent costly reinjury.

Prevention of Secondary Complications

Interventions focused on prevention are within the scope of skilled occupational therapy if it can be shown that the client has a high risk of developing complications. Secondary complications might include prevention of progressive joint contractures, fracture nonunion, and skin breakdown. Other prevention programs and strategies might include early intervention programs, drug/alcohol relapse prevention programs, assessment of ergonomics in the workplace, instruction in joint protection, energy conservation, and provision of wellness programs.

The AOTA website (www.aota.org) contains a section on reimbursement and regulatory policy that is very helpful in determining what occupational therapy services are reimbursable.

Billing Codes

Since 1983, reimbursement for many health care services has been based on the Diagnostic Related Groups (DRGs) and the codes into which problems and services are classified. There are two primary coding systems currently used: (1) *The International Classification of Diseases* (ICD) codes and (2) the *Physician's Current Procedural Terminology* (CPT) codes (Contant, 2003).

ICD-9 and ICD-10 Codes

The International Classification of Diseases was developed by the WHO. ICD-9 refers to the 9th edition of the ICD codes, which is currently in use in the United States, although ICD-10 has been implemented for reporting mortality (Olson, 2004). The ICD-9 codes classify diagnoses, symptoms, or complaints, and serve as a basis for determining DRGs (Contant, 2003). These are 3, 4, or 5 digit codes. Some codes are complete at 4 digits, and some go to 5 digits. For example, 710 through 739 apply to diseases of the musculoskeletal system and connective tissue, and 728.87 is the ICD-9 code for muscle weakness. The ICD codes are often used to support medical necessity (Olson 2004). Code books may be purchased from a variety of sources, including the U.S. Government Printing Office, and training in basic ICD-9 coding is available free from the Centers for Medicare and Medicaid Services (CMS) learning website at http://www.cms.hhs.gov/medlearn/therapy.

CPT Codes

Current Procedural Terminology (CPT) codes were first published by the American Medical Association in 1966, and are revised yearly effective every January first. These are numeric 5 digit codes that are copyrighted by the American Medical Association (Olson, 2004). The goal of the CPT codes is establishment of a common language when submitting claims for billing services provided by physicians and other health care providers. Some codes are time based (broken into 15-minute time periods) and others are "procedures," which are billed at the same amount regardless of how much time is used (Olson, 2004). For example, 97003 is the CPT code for occupational therapy evaluation, which is considered a procedure. Some codes are "bundled", or are mutually exclusive. For example, an OT evaluation may not be billed along with a manual muscle test, since the manual muscle test is considered a part of the evaluation. Facilities often provide a list of the most commonly used codes (Gennerman, 2005). Code books may be purchased from a variety of sources, and CPT codes are also published on the CMS website.

Recipients of Occupational Therapy Services

Individuals served by occupational therapists and occupational therapy assistants are most often referred to as **clients**. The *Occupational Therapy Practice Framework* (AOTA, 2002) tells us that this term is:

> Consistent with the *Guide to Occupational Therapy Practice* (Moyers, 1999) and indicative of the profession's growing understanding that people may be served not only as individuals, but also as members of a group or a population. The actual term used for individuals who are served will vary by practice setting. For example, in a hospital the person might be referred to as a *patient*, whereas in a school he or she might be called a *student* (p. 615).

Note: In this manual, the terms client, patient, student, child, infant, consumer, resident, individual, veteran, and first names have been used to reflect the terms used in various practice settings. Names have been fabricated to protect the confidentiality of those people who receive our services. In a note that says "Mr. P. was seen in his home....." please understand that he is being called "Mr. P." for purposes of confidentiality. If you were writing a note in his health record, you would use his whole name.

Overview

The information in this manual has been arranged in the order that it is most easily learned, with the more straightforward concepts being offered first. More complex concepts build on these as clinical reasoning is developed. Chapter 2: The Health Record provides an introduction to the medical (health) record—its function, uses, and history. The history of the SOAP note is included, along with the mechanics of writing in the record. Also included in Chapter 2 is a brief list of standard abbreviations and symbols that may be used in completing the exercises in this manual.

Chapter 3: Writing Functional Problem Statements discusses the mechanics of writing problem statements. After you evaluate a client, you develop a problem list, which is essentially a list of those areas of occupation that you think you can impact positively with occupational therapy intervention strategies. From this list, you formulate **functional problem statements**. After the problems have been defined and prioritized, goals are formulated with the client. The goals are worded in behavioral and measurable terms. This includes both long-term goals (**goals**) and short-term goals (**objectives**). Chapter 4: Writing Functional and Measurable Goals and Objectives discusses the format for writing goals and objectives. Worksheets are provided for practice, and some examples of problem and goal statements offer you help if you are having trouble.

The following four chapters teach the four sections of the SOAP format (Subjective, Objective, Assessment, and Plan), which have been introduced and explained in Chapters 1 and 2. Multiple examples are presented for each section, and worksheets are provided for practice. Following the chapters that teach basic skills, intervention planning is discussed in Chapter 9: Intervention Planning, since the intervention plan is a vital part of the initial evaluation.

Chapter 10: Documenting Different Stages of Treatment discusses the different kinds of notes that are written at different stages of the treatment process. From the first notation in the chart that a referral has been received to the closing lines of the discontinuation summary, occupational therapists and occupational therapy assistants document the many and varied activities of the intervention process. The specific content of the note, the format of the note, and the time lines required vary according to type of setting, accrediting and regulatory agencies involved, and requirements of third party payers. The contents required for each type of note are described in *Guidelines for Documentation of Occupational Therapy* (AOTA, 2003). We will address the requirements for the following kinds of notes.

Initial Evaluation Reports

Before beginning treatment, the occupational therapist evaluates the client to determine whether occupational therapy is appropriate for this client, and if so, what kind of therapeutic intervention will be most useful. Each setting has its own way of evaluating a client. A mental health center, for example, may not do the same kind of initial evaluation as a public school or a skilled nursing facility. Initial evaluations are usually documented on forms provided by the setting, but may also be done in a SOAP format.

Contact Notes

Each time an intervention is provided by the occupational therapist, notation is made of what occurred. Contacts may also include telephone calls and meetings with other people. In some settings, each treatment session is documented in the health record using a contact note. In other settings, the therapist keeps a log or makes notes to himself for use later in writing progress notes, but no formalized contact note is required. Many different formats are used for writing contact notes, but in this manual the SOAP format will be taught.

Progress Notes

At the end of a specified period of time, a progress note is written documenting the client's progress toward goals and detailing any changes made in the intervention plan. Different practice settings use different time periods for reporting, usually weekly or monthly. Progress notes may also be written in different formats, but will be taught in a SOAP format in this manual.

Reevaluation Notes

The reevaluation that is part of the occupational therapy intervention process may be documented in a formal reevaluation report in some settings. For example, in a practice setting where managed care is involved, a client may need to be reevaluated in order to be recertified for treatment after the number of visits initially allocated are completed.

Transition Notes

Transition notes are written when a client is transferring from one service setting to another, such as from acute care to rehabilitation or from rehabilitation to skilled nursing. Transition notes insure that the client's intervention plan remains intact through the move, and that services that have already been provided are not duplicated.

Discharge or Discontinuation Notes

At the end of treatment, a discharge note is written to describe changes in the client's ability to engage in meaningful occupation as a result of occupational therapy intervention. Discharge notes summarize the course of treatment, progress toward goals, status at the time of discharge, any home program that may have been recommended, and any other recommendations or referrals. Some settings provide a specific form for the discharge note and other facilities may use the same form that was used for the evaluation. For purposes of this manual, a SOAP format will be used.

Chapter 11: Documentation in Different Practice Settings discusses the special requirements of different kinds of practice settings (mental health, long-term care, school-based practice, palliative care, and consultation), and Chapter 12: Making Good Notes Even Better begins with a review of what you have learned, and then takes your skills to the next level. Notes from a variety of treatment settings are provided at the end of the manual in Chapter 13: Examples of Different Kinds of Notes, in addition to the examples scattered throughout the book. The Appendix (Suggestions for Completing the Worksheets) provides "answers" for the worksheets. However, since there are many "right" ways to answer, these must be viewed as suggestions rather than the only "correct" answers.

New in This Edition

The second edition of *Documentation Manual for Writing SOAP Notes in Occupational Therapy* is based on the *Occupational Therapy Practice Framework* (AOTA, 2002a) and on the *Guidelines for Documentation of Occupational Therapy* (AOTA, 2003). The second edition includes a brief introduction to billing codes and HIPAA. In addition, the examples used in the text and the worksheets are more diverse, with increased examples from psychiatric and pediatric practice settings, as well as a few examples of palliative care and complementary therapy. Some chapters have been reorganized to make the material easier to understand, and worksheets have been added to teach concepts that were confusing to some readers in the first edition. Chapter 12 has been expanded to take documentation skills to the next level.

Roles of the Registered Occupational Therapist and Certified Occupational Therapy Assistant

Occupational therapists (OTs) and occupational therapy assistants (OTAs) have different roles and responsibilities in documenting the occupational therapy intervention process. In its *Guidelines for Supervision, Roles, and Responsibilities During the Delivery of Occupational Therapy Services,* AOTA provides very specific guidelines for roles and responsibilities of both OTs and OTAs in documentation (AOTA, 2004a). The OTA collaborates with the OT in designing, implementing, and assessing occupational therapy services. The OTA may contribute to documentation at all stages of treatment under the supervision of the OT and concurring with relevant laws and regulations (AOTA, 2004a).

Although these guidelines are considered "best practice," state statutes may differ from the guidelines. The guidelines may also differ from federal laws that delineate mandatory documentation requirements. Sometimes reimbursement organizations specify who would be an approved documenter for reimbursement purposes. You as a therapist are accountable for adhering to the mandatory policies and procedures adopted by state and federal regulatory agencies, but you will find the standards established by AOTA useful in interpreting and following regulations.

Conclusion

In the following pages you will be introduced to the health record and to the specifics of your documentation in the record. There will be ample explanation and opportunity for practice, so that in the end **you** will be the occupational therapist we talked about in the beginning paragraph whose documentation was so amazing to the beginning student.

Chapter 2
THE HEALTH RECORD

Definition and Purpose

The health record (sometimes called the medical record) is a compilation of data that includes the client's past and present health information. The purpose of the record is documentation of the client's condition and treatment, particularly the current episode (Pickett, 2003). Like so many other aspects of health care, the health record is undergoing vast changes as we move further into the information age. Although the record is the physical property of the facility that compiles it, individuals have a right to review and obtain a copy of their records, except in certain specified circumstances (United States Department of Health and Human Services, 2003).

History

Health care can be traced back approximately 7000 years to early medicine men who were thought to be able to communicate with the spirit world. Written records can be found as early as 2700 B.C. in Egypt (Abdelhak, Grostick, Hanken, & Jacobs, 2001). After one of the first hospitals in America was incorporated in Pennsylvania in 1792, its secretary, Benjamin Franklin, began to keep records of clients' names, addresses, disorders, and dates of admission and discharge. These early records were often kept in ledgers, and were brief and handwritten. As medicine advanced, so did the complexity and detail of the record. A profession (now called Health Information Management) was created to oversee the record.

The increasing mobility of people and the shift from primarily local health care delivery organizations to regional and national enterprises has created a need for more sophisticated health information systems (Mancilla, 2003). The electronic health record is designed to allow clinicians easy access to complete and accurate data upon which to base clinical decisions, even if these clinicians are in different locations. However, rapid access must be balanced against the security and integrity of the record, leaving a number of sticky and as yet unanswered questions (Abdelhak, et al., 2001).

The Problem-Oriented Medical Record

The problem-oriented medical record (POMR) was introduced in the 1960s by Lawrence Weed, a physician who wanted to provide a more client-centered approach to the structure of the record (Kiger, 2003). He saw the record as being arranged for the convenience of the staff, rather than ordered for the highest good of the client and suggested that the record be organized into four sections:

1. A database, containing the history and physical, evaluations by all disciplines, lab results, etc.
2. A list of the client's problems.
3. An interdisciplinary treatment plan, developed by all the clinicians working with the client.
4. Progress notes written in chronological order, regardless of discipline.

By organizing the chart in this manner, there is a focus on the client's problems and the progress toward the solution to those problems, avoiding the fragmentation of the source-oriented record (Kiger, 2003). There is no need to search the chart to see what each discipline has to say about a particular area of concern. The progress notes are also integrated, rather than being organized by discipline, so that all the information regarding what has happened for/to the client on that day is in one place. In this way, it is easy for any member of the health care team to read progress notes for the last 24 hours and know everything that is current without having to search several sections of the chart for the necessary information.

As a part of the more client-centered approach to documentation, Weed recommended that the progress note be organized into four sections including the client's own perception of the situation, which had heretofore been considered irrelevant. These four sections included:

S (Subjective): The client's perception of the treatment being received, the progress, limitations, needs, and problems. Normally the subjective section of the note is brief. In an initial evaluation note, however, the "S" might be longer, since it will contain the information obtained in the initial interview.

O (Objective): The health professional's observations of the treatment being provided. In an initial evaluation note, this section also contains of all the measurable, quantifiable, and observable data that were collected. In an evaluation, the first two sections form the database from which a problem list and treatment plan evolve. Some facilities have combined the first two sections into a composite category called data and have adapted Weed's SOAP notes into DAP notes. For purposes of this manual, we will continue to use the two discrete sections.

A (Assessment): The health professional's interpretation of the meaning of the events reported in the objective section. This section includes functional limitations, along with expectations of the client's ability to benefit from therapy (sometimes called rehabilitation potential). An initial evaluation also contains the problem list, which is one of the key elements of the POMR method of charting. In a progress note, the assessment component contains an explicit statement of progress or the lack of progress. In a POMR, each progress note is tied to a problem from the client's problem list. That problem is stated at the beginning of the note.

P (Plan): What the health professional plans to do next to continue with the goals and objectives in the intervention plan. In an initial evaluation, this section contains the intervention plan along with the anticipated frequency and duration of treatment.

For almost 30 years, Weed's system was popular in hospitals and rehabilitation centers. Gradually, however, many facilities have returned to a more source-oriented medical record, containing sections for each discipline. Even so, the SOAP format of progress notes has remained popular in facilities that no longer use the POMR.

Remember that SOAP is just a format — an outline for organizing information. Any note can be written in this format, although some notes lend themselves to it better than others. For example, you could write an initial assessment in a SOAP format, or a discharge summary, contact note, reassessment or progress note. An initial assessment can be quite lengthy when written this way, as it will contain an occupational profile, a summary of functional problems, short- and long-term goals, prior level of functioning, and the beginning intervention plan. For this reason, most practice settings would not use the SOAP format for the initial evaluation report, even if that facility used SOAP for its treatment and progress notes.

The SOAP format is an alternative to narrative notes, which tend to be disorganized and subjective. It forces the writer to look at all four aspects of the intervention session, and to present the information contained in the note in an orderly fashion. A more detailed discussion of each section of the note follows in Chapters 5 through 8.

Health Insurance Portability and Accountancy Act (HIPAA)

In 1996, Congress passed the Health Insurance Portability and Accountancy Act (HIPAA), which was implemented in 1998. One of the missions of HIPAA is the protection of personal health information from inappropriate access, modification, or use (Mancilla, 2003). HIPAA establishes national standards for the security, use, and disclosure of a client's health information, as well as standards for a client's right to understand and control how their health information is used (United States Department of Health and Human Services, 2003). In very practical terms, this means not leaving records open on a desk or up on a screen where they can be read by others (Sames, 2005).

Users and Uses of the Health Record

The health record is a communication tool, and as such it has many different uses and users. It is important to consider all your different audiences when you make an entry in the client's record.

Client Care Management

The record is one of the ways the treatment team communicates with each other about the day-to-day aspects of a client's care. Other therapists in your own department or members of the treatment team will read your notes in order to coordinate care. In your note you share the results of your evaluation, report your client's progress toward established goals, and advise other members of the team of your plan for continuing care, all of which are important to the treatment team. In a situation where occupational therapy is provided 7 days per week, one occupational therapist may not be providing all of the client's care and may depend upon the treatment notes to find out what treatment was provided in his or her absence.

Reimbursement

The health record is the source document for what services were provided, and thus, for what services may be billed. It is used in billing to substantiate reimbursement claims. For example, if there were a question about the duration and frequency of interventions provided, the record would be the source document used to answer that question.

The Legal System

The health record is a legal document that substantiates what occurred during a client's illness/treatment. If you as an occupational therapist have to appear in court to testify, you will be very glad that your documentation is clear and thorough. Sometimes court cases occur years after the event or intervention that is being contested. You may not even remember the event or the client. What you have written in the health record will provide you with the information you need in order to testify.

Quality Improvement

Most facilities have a Quality Improvement (QI) Committee whose duty is to oversee the adequacy and appropriateness of the care that is being provided. This committee is in charge of finding and solving problems in client care. The health record is one of the primary sources of information used in the QI process.

Research

The record is also used to provide data for medical research. Some research uses individual data specific to that client while other research uses aggregate data where no client name is attached to the data. In either case, the source document is often the health record, under the security regulations of HIPAA.

Accreditation

Accrediting agencies such as the Centers for Medicare and Medicaid (CMS) and the Commission on Accreditation of Rehabilitation Facilities (CARF) review your notes to ascertain whether the extent and quality of services provided by your facility and/or your department meet the standards of care set by the accrediting agency. If your facility is found not in compliance, accreditation may be withdrawn. For example, the CMS accredits facilities that bill for Medicare. If the facility does not meet CMS standards, all claims made by that facility for Medicare services will be denied. The health record is one of the primary sources of information used during an accreditation visit.

Education

The record may be used as a teaching tool. A student uses the health record to gain information about clients and about quality and appropriate occupational therapy intervention, in accord with the security regulations of HIPAA.

Public Health

The record is also used to identify and to document the incidence of certain diseases, such as tuberculosis or HIV.

Utilization Management

In a hospital setting, the Utilization Review Committee is charged with determining how services in the facility are being utilized, that is, what kinds of clients are being seen and what kind of care is being provided, and whether these are appropriate to the mission of the facility.

Business Development

Management teams use the information contained in the record to plan and market the services provided by the facility. For example, are enough cases of eating disorder being admitted to open a special eating disorders unit?

The Client

Another significant user is the client. When you are writing in the health record, always remember that the client owns the information in his or her own record and may choose to exercise his or her right to read what you have written.

Writing in the Record

Since the health record is not only a communication tool during the client's hospital stay, but is also the source document for financial, legal, and clinical accountability, the record should show the following:
- What services were provided and when.
- What happened and what was said.
- How the client responded to the service provided.
- Why your skill as an OT was needed rather than the services of an aide or family member.

Before you write anything in the record, make these assumptions:
- Someone else will have to read and understand what I write because I may be sick or out of town the next time this client needs to be treated.
- This entry I am about to make will be the one scrutinized by a CMS review team or a Blue Cross representative. If I were a funding source, would I want to pay for the services I am about to record?
- My client will exercise his or her right to read this record.

As discussed in Chapter 1, it is critical to know your payment sources when documenting. Some payers are looking for quite different outcomes than others. With a Medicare client, you will discuss activities of daily living (ADLs) and write goals for self-care activities. With a workers' compensation case, you will write goals that are oriented to return to work. With home care, you may need to document that your client is unable to leave home to receive services or that education on safety issues was provided to the caregiver. With a child, you will need to focus on developmental needs or educationally related services identified in the Individualized Education Plan (IEP).

Also remember these facts when planning to write in a client's record:

- Accuracy is your best protection against problems. You cannot be accurate if you wait too long to record what happened.
- A note in the health record is going to be a reflection of your professional identity and abilities as well as a reflection of your department and occupational therapy as a profession.
- No activity or contact is ever considered a service that has been provided until a clinical entry is in the record. In terms of fiscal and legal accountability, "If it isn't written, it didn't happen."

Helpful hints on writing notes:
- Be as concise as possible without leaving out pertinent data.
- Avoid generalities.
- Report behavior and avoid judgments except in assessing your data.
- Be sparse with technical jargon that may be unfamiliar to the reader.

The Mechanics of Documentation

There are a few "rules" that must be followed when writing in the record:

1. *Always use waterproof black ink.*
   After a certain period of time, health records are microfilmed, and black ink is the only color that microfilms adequately.
2. *Never use white out.*
   Using white out in a health record is considered illegally altering the record. The health record is a legal document that must stand as originally written.
3. *Correct errors.*
   If you make an error in the health record, draw one line through it, write your correction, and initial the change:

   SB

   Pt. able to dress lower body with ~~verbal cues~~ min Ⓐ using a reacher.

   In a problem-oriented medical chart, if you inadvertently write your note in the wrong client's chart, draw a single line through the entire entry and write "wrong chart" beside it with your signature.
   If you need to add something after you have written and signed your note, write an addendum with the current date and time.
4. *Be sure all required data is present.*
   The *Guidelines for Documentation of Occupational Therapy* (AOTA, 2003) specify the contents for each type of note you may be writing. This information will be covered in Chapter 10. Make certain that your note contains all the necessary information, and remember, it is absolutely critical that you date and sign your note. The standard of signature is first name, middle initial if available, last name, and credentials. Some settings require a printed name and credentials beneath the signature (Olson, 2004).

5.   *Be concise.*
      In today's health care system, busy professionals are often pressed for time and appreci-
      ate being able to read what you have written in the shortest time possible. Your own
      time for documentation will also be limited under today's productivity standards.
6.   *Use appropriate terminology for the recipients of services.*
      When referring to the persons who use occupational therapy services, we may use
      the terms client, patient, consumer, resident, veteran, participant, individual, student,
      teacher, employer, family, or administrator. Please use the term that is considered most
      respectful in your practice setting.
7.   *Be prudent in using abbreviations.*
      Use only the abbreviations that are approved by your facility. While it saves time to use
      symbols and abbreviations, remember that your notes may be read by someone who
      knows little about occupational therapy and who will determine whether or not to pay
      for your services. It is wise to be sure that the person is able to understand what you
      have written. Your facility will be able to furnish a list of the abbreviations it allows so
      that the abbreviations and symbols that you use will be validated if there is a question.
      Do not make up your own abbreviations, and do not use any abbreviation that is not
      on your facility's approved list. Remember, it is permitted to use abbreviations, but it is
      not necessary. You are permitted to write out any word instead of shortening it. In this
      manual you will find that some notes use more abbreviations and symbols than others.

Using Medical Terminology

The Joint Commission on the Accreditation of Health Care Organizations (JCAHO), which
accredits hospitals and other health care facilities, does not maintain a list of acceptable abbreviations
and symbols for use in documentation, although it does maintain a list of those that are prohibited.
JCAHO encourages clinicians to write out words rather than relying on abbreviations and symbols.
When in doubt, refer to the JCAHO website at www.jcaho.org.

In order to maintain uniformity and clarity in the health record, each health care facility
establishes a list of approved abbreviations and symbols that clinicians may use in documentation.
For purposes of using this manual, the list of abbreviations in Table 2-1 will be permitted.

TABLE 2-1

Abbreviations and Symbols

A	anterior; assessment
AA	Alcoholics Anonymous
Ⓐ	assistance
$\bar{a}$	before
AAROM	active assistive range of motion
abd	abduction
ABI	acquired brain injury
add	adduction
ADD	Attention Deficit Disorder
ADHD	Attention Deficit Hyperactivity Disorder
ADL	activity of daily living
ad lib.	as desired
AE	above elbow
AIDS	acquired immunodeficiency syndrome
AK	above knee
AKA	above knee amputation
am, AM	morning
AMA	against medical advice
AMB	ambulation
amt.	amount
AP	anterior-posterior
AROM	active range of motion
ASAP	as soon as possible
ASHD	arteriosclerotic heart disease
ASIS	anterior superior iliac spine
Ⓑ	bilateral
BADL	basic activity of daily living
BE	below elbow
b.i.d.	twice a day
BK	below knee
BKA	below knee amputation
BM	black male; bowel movement
BP	blood pressure
BRP	bathroom privileges
$\bar{c}$	with
C	Celsius; centigrade
CA	carcinoma; cancer
C&S	culture and sensitivity
CABG	coronary artery bypass graft
CAT	computerized axial tomography
CBC	complete blood count
CCU	coronary (cardiac) care unit
CGA	contact guard assist
CHF	congestive heart failure
CHI	closed head injury
CHT	certified hand therapist
cm	centimeter
CNS	central nervous system
CO_2	carbon dioxide

TABLE 2-1 (CONTINUED)

Abbreviations and Symbols

C/O	complains of
CMC	carpometacarpal
cont.	continue
COPD	chronic obstructive pulmonary disease
COTA	certified occupational therapy assistant
CP	cerebral palsy
CPR	cardiopulmonary resuscitation
CSF	cerebrospinal fluid
CST	craniosacral therapist
CT	computed tomography
CTR	carpal tunnel release
CVA	cerebrovascular accident
CXR	chest x-ray
d̲	day
Ⓓ	dependent
D&C	dilation and curettage
D.D.S.	doctor of dental surgery
DIP	distal interphalangeal joint
DJD	degenerative joint disease
DLS	daily living skills
DM	diabetes mellitus
DME	durable medical equipment
D.O.	doctor of osteopathic medicine
DOB	date of birth
Dr.	doctor
DRG	diagnostic related group
DTR	deep tendon reflex
DVT	deep vein thrombosis
Dx	diagnosis
ECG	electrocardiogram
ECHO	echocardiogram
EEG	electroencephalogram
EKG	electrocardiogram
EMG	electromyogram
ENT	ear, nose, throat
EOB	edge of bed
ER	emergency room
etc.	etcetera
ETOH	ethyl alcohol
eval.	evaluation
ext.	extension
F	Fahrenheit; fair (muscle strength grade of 3)
f	female
F.A.C.P.	fellow of the American College of Physicians
F.A.C.S.	fellow of the American College of Surgeons
FBS	fasting blood sugar
flex.	flexion
fl oz	fluid ounce

TABLE 2-1 (CONTINUED)

Abbreviations and Symbols

FROM	functional range of motion
ft.	foot, feet (the measurement, not the body part)
FWB	full weight bearing
Fx	fracture
G	good (muscle strength grade of 4)
GB	gallbladder
GI	gastrointestinal
gm	gram
GYN	gynecology
h	hour
HA, H/A	headache
HH	home health
H&P	history and physical
HBV	hepatitis B virus
HEENT	head, eyes, ears, nose, throat
HEP	home exercise program
HIV	human immunodeficiency virus
HOB	head of bed
HOH	hand over hand
HR	heart rate
hr.	hour
HRT	hormone replacement therapy
Ht	height
HTN	hypertension
Hx	history
Ⓘ	independent
IADL	instrumental activity of daily living
i.e.	that is
ICU	intensive care unit
IM	intramuscular
IMP	impression
in.	inches
int.	internal
IP	inpatient
ITP	individualized treatment plan
IUD	intrauterine device
IV	intravenous
kg	kilogram
Ⓛ	left
lb.	pound
LE	lower extremity
LLQ	left lower quadrant
LRTI	ligament reconstruction tendinous interposition
LTG	long-term goal
LUQ	left upper quadrant
m	murmur; meter; male
max	maximum
meds.	medications

TABLE 2-1 (CONTINUED)

Abbreviations and Symbols

MD	muscular dystrophy; medical doctor
MFT	muscle function test
MI	myocardial infarction
min	minutes; minimum
mm	millimeter
MME	(Folstein's) Mini-Mental Status Examination
MMT	manual muscle test
mo.	month
mod	moderate
MP, MCP	metacarpophalangeal
MRI	magnetic resonance imaging
MVA	motor vehicle accident
N	normal (muscle strength grade of 5)
NDT	neurodevelopmental treatment
neg.	negative
NG	nasogastric
NICU	neonatal intensive care unit
NKA	no known allergy
NKDA	no known drug allergy
noc.	night
NPO	nothing by mouth
NSR	normal sinus rhythm
NWB	non-weight bearing
O	objective; oriented
O_2	oxygen
OX4	oriented to time, place, person, situation
OB	obstetrics
OBS	organic brain syndrome
OP	outpatient
OR	operating room
ORIF	open reduction, internal fixation
OT	occupational therapist; occupational therapy
oz	ounce
$\bar{p}$	after
P	plan; posterior; pulse; poor (muscle strength grade of 2)
PA	posterior anterior; physician's assistant
PADL	personal activity of daily living
PAP	Papanicolaou test (smear)
PDD	Pervasive Developmental Disorder
PE	physical examination
per	by
peri.	perineal
PET	positron emission tomography
Ph.D.	doctor of philosophy
PIP	proximal interphalangeal
PLOF	prior level of functioning
pm, PM	afternoon
PNF	proprioceptive neuromuscular facilitation

TABLE 2-1 (CONTINUED)

Abbreviations and Symbols

PNI	peripheral nerve injury
PNS	peripheral nervous system
p.o.	by mouth
POMR	problem-oriented medical record
pos.	positive
poss.	possible
post op	post operation
pre op	pre operation
p.r.n.	as needed
pro	pronation
PROM	passive range of motion
pt.	patient
PT	physical therapist; physical therapy
PTA	physical therapist assistant; prior to admission
PWB	partial weight bearing
Px	physical examination
q	every
q.i.d.	four times a day
qt.	quart
R̄	respiration
Ⓡ	right
RA	rheumatoid arthritis
RBC	red blood cell count
R.D.	registered dietician
re:	regarding
rehab	rehabilitation
resp	respiratory; respiration
R.Ph.	registered pharmacist
RLQ	right lower quadrant
R/O	rule out
ROM	range of motion
ROS	review of symptoms
RROM	resistive range of motion
R.T.	respiratory therapist; recreation therapist
RTC	return to clinic
RTO	return to office
RUQ	right upper quadrant
RSD	reflex sympathetic dystrophy
Rx	recipe; Latin *take thou prescription*
s̄	without
S	subjective
SBA	stand by assistance
SH	social history
Sig:	instruction to patient
SLE	systemic lupus erythematosus
SOC	start of care

TABLE 2-1 (CONTINUED)
Abbreviations and Symbols

SNF	skilled nursing facility
SOAP	subjective, objective, assessment, plan
SOB	shortness of breath
S/P	status post
STAT	immediately
STD	sexually transmitted disease
STG	short-term goal
STM	short-term memory
sup	supination
suppos	suppository
Sx	symptom
T	temperature; trace (muscle strength grade of 1)
TB	tuberculosis
TBI	traumatic brain injury
tbsp.	tablespoon
TEDS	thrombo-embolic disease stockings
TENS	transcutaneous electrical nerve stimulator (also TNS)
THR	total hip replacement
TIA	transient ischemic attack
t.i.d.	three times a day
TKR	total knee replacement
TM(J)	temporomandibular (joint)
TNR	tonic neck reflex (also ATNR; STNR)
t.o.	telephone order
TPR	temperature, pulse, & respiration
TRS	therapeutic recreation specialist
tx.	treatment; traction
UA	urinalysis
UE	upper extremity
UMN	upper motor neuron
URI	upper respiratory infection
US	ultrasound
UTI	urinary tract infection
UV	ultraviolet
VC	vital capacity
VD	venereal disease
v.o.	verbal orders
vol.	volume
VS	vital signs
WBC	white blood cell; white blood count
w/c	wheelchair
WDWN	well developed, well nourished
WFL	within functional limits
wk.	week
WNL	within normal limits
wt	weight
x or X	times

TABLE 2-1 (CONTINUED)

Abbreviations and Symbols

y.o.	year old
yd.	yard
yr.	year

Symbols

x1, x2	assistance (assistance of 1 person given; also written "assistance of 1") *Example*: "transferred to toilet c̄ min Ⓐ x2"
♂	male
♀	female
↓	down; downward; decrease
↑	up; upward; increase
c	with
s̄	without
p̄	after
ā	before
~	approximately
@	at
Δ	change
>	greater than
<	less than
=	equals
+	plus; positive (also abbreviated pos.)
–	minus; negative (also abbreviated neg.)
#	number (#1); pounds
/	per
%	percent
&	and
°	degree
↔	to and from
→	to; progressing forward; approaching
1°	primary
2°	secondary; secondary to
"	inches
'	feet

WORKSHEET 2-1
Using Abbreviations

Translate each sentence written with abbreviations into full English phrases or sentences.

Client c/o pain in Ⓡ MCP joint $\bar{p}$ ~ 15 min PROM.

Client w/c → mat $\bar{c}$ sliding board max Ⓐ x2.

Pt. O x 4.

1° dx. THR 2° dx. COPD & CHF.

Shorten these notes using only the standard abbreviations in this chapter:

Client has thirty degrees of passive range of motion in the left distal interphalangeal joint which is within functional limits.

Client is able to put on her socks with standby assistance, but requires moderate assistance with putting on and taking off left shoe.

The client requires contact guard assistance for balance during her morning dressing which she performs while sitting on the edge of her bed.

WORKSHEET 2-2
Additional Practice

Shorten these notes using only the standard abbreviations in this chapter:

The patient was seen bedside for evaluation of activities of daily living. She was able to perform bed mobility exercises with moderate assistance, but needed maximum assistance to put on her adult undergarment. She was able to go from a supine position to a sitting position with minimum assistance and from a sitting position to a standing position with moderate assistance.

The resident came to the occupational therapy clinic via wheelchair escort. The resident was observed to lean to his left. The resident needed verbal cues and minimum assistance in positioning his body in the wheelchair to maintain midline orientation and symmetrical posture. The resident transferred from his wheelchair to the toilet with moderate assistance of one person to help him keep his balance using a standing pivot transfer. He needed verbal cues and visual feedback from a mirror to maintain upright posture.

The veteran was seen in his own room seated in a wheelchair for an evaluation of relevant client factors. The veteran's short-term memory was three out of three for immediate recall, one out of three after 1 minute, and zero out of three with verbal cues after 5 minutes. The left upper extremity shoulder flexion was a grade of 4, shoulder extension was a grade of 4, elbow flexion was a grade of 4, elbow extension was a grade of 4, wrist extension was a grade of 4 minus, wrist flexion was a grade of 4 minus, and grip strength was 8 pounds. The left upper extremity light touch is intact. The right upper extremity muscle grades and sensation are within functional limits.

From Borcherding S. *Documentation Manual for Writing SOAP Notes in Occupational Therapy, Second Edition.*
© 2005 SLACK Incorporated

Chapter 3
WRITING FUNCTIONAL PROBLEM STATEMENTS

As a part of the initial assessment, the occupational therapist develops a "problem list" identifying the major areas of occupation and underlying factors that are not within functional limits (WFL). Priorities are then set with the client and family so that the problems that are most important to them will be addressed. Some clients will be able to identify problem areas easily, while others may not understand occupational therapy well and it may need to be explained to the client in a meaningful way (Kannenberg & Greene, 2003).

The diagnosis is *not* the problem. For example, if the client has sustained a head injury, the problem is *not* TBI, but rather the areas of occupation that are no longer WFL such as,

Client is unable to carry out personal ADL tasks due to <45 second attention span.

Client needs mod Ⓐ in dressing due to poor trunk stability.

Areas of Occupation

In writing problem statements, we will include two important items: the area of occupation that is a concern, and the factors that are interfering with the client's engagement in that area of occupation. As noted in Chapter 1, there are seven areas of occupation identified in the *Framework*. These are:

1. Activities of daily living (basic or personal)
2. Instrumental activities of daily living
3. Education
4. Work
5. Play
6. Leisure
7. Social participation

As occupational therapists, we recognize that a client's sense of well-being depends partly on the ability to participate in the life roles desired at home, at work, at school, and in the community. It is the inability to participate in roles or activities or situations as desired that constitute problems, rather than the diagnosis or physical impairment itself. Thus we might see problem statements such as these:

- Child needs mod Ⓐ to hold scissors to complete art activities in school.
- Fear of leaving the house limits client's ability to participate in social events in the community.
- Veteran requires mod Ⓐ in transfer to toilet due to trunk instability.
- Three steps leading to front door limit Andy's ability to enter his home.

Note that each of these statements identifies the **area of occupation** (school, social participation, ADL) that is problematic for the client. Some of the seven areas are considered medically necessary by third party payers and some are not, and we will factor that information into writing our problem statements also.

Underlying Factors

The second part of the problem statement identifies the underlying factor that is limiting engagement in the desired occupation, role, or activity. Underlying factors may include performance skills or patterns, contexts, activity demands, and client factors (AOTA, 2000). Let's look at some of these underlying factors.

Performance Skills

Performance skills are the units that make up an activity. Motor skills such as the ability to move the fingers into tripod pinch, process skills such as the ability to sequence a task, and communication skills such as the ability to answer a question are all performance skills.

Performance Patterns

Performance patterns are habits, routines, or roles that we don't usually think about. Patterns may be helpful ways of going through the day, such as a morning routine for grooming and dressing, or they may be destructive routines that need to be changed, such as the rituals and patterns around alcohol and drug use.

Context

Context may include not only place, but also such things as time, space, age, social factors, or even internal things such as beliefs. In writing problem and goal statements, we need to consider the context in which the client might wish to participate.

Activity Demands

Activity demands are the different pieces of the task that are required to carry out the activity. For example, to engage in a writing task you would need a pencil, some way to grasp the pencil, motor coordination, and some ability to sequence. All of those are demands of a writing activity.

Client Factors

Client factors include body structures and body functions. Low vision, high muscle tone, and hallucinations are all examples of client factors.

For a complete discussion of the underlying factors that comprise problems in occupational functioning, please refer to the *Occupational Therapy Practice Framework: Domain and Process* (AOTA, 2002a).

WORKSHEET 3-1
Identifying the Underlying Factors

Now let us try building a problem statement. First we will begin with an area of occupation. In the first case, we will use work as our area of occupation.

Consumer is unable to sustain employment longer than 2 weeks due to....

This problem statement needs to be completed with the underlying factor that is causing difficulty. Perhaps your client is unable to sustain attention long enough to complete a work task. Perhaps instead there is a problem with reliable transportation. These are very different problem areas, requiring very different interventions.

In the space below, complete this problem statement with at least three possible limiting factors, not including the examples given above.

Consumer is unable to sustain employment longer than 2 weeks due to

Consumer is unable to sustain employment longer than 2 weeks due to

Consumer is unable to sustain employment longer than 2 weeks due to

Now consider the second problem statement, with personal ADL as its area of occupation:

Veteran needs 1½ hours to complete grooming activities due to

In the space below, complete this problem statement with three possible underlying factors:

Veteran needs 1½ hours to complete grooming activities due to

Veteran needs 1½ hours to complete grooming activities due to

Veteran needs 1½ hours to complete grooming activities due to

In formulating problem statements, be sure the problem identified is one that will respond to OT treatment. There is no need to identify problems you do not intend to treat.

From Borcherding S. *Documentation Manual for Writing SOAP Notes in Occupational Therapy, Second Edition.*
© 2005 SLACK Incorporated

Writing Problem Statements

Now let's look at some formulas or protocols for writing problem statements. You will need three components in your problem statement:

1. An area of occupation.
2. An underlying factor to be treated in occupational therapy.
3. *If possible,* a measuring device for the underlying factor.

The following problem statements use an assist level as the measuring device.

Client requires mod assist to don pants 2° 3+ upper extremity strength.

Child needs mod Ⓐ to hold scissors to complete art activities in school due to immature grasp pattern.

Jody requires mod verbal cues to stay on task during school activities 2° to attention span of <5 minutes.

Consumer needs mod verbal cues to remember to make eye contact during social interactions.

For ease of writing, you can use the following formula to write a problem statement:

Client needs _____ in _____ due to _____.
           Assist level   Performing what occupational task   underlying factor

For example:

Child needs mod Ⓐ to hold scissors to complete art activities in school due to high tone.

Veteran requires mod Ⓐ in transfer to toilet due to trunk instability.

The use of a measuring tool is helpful in documenting progress toward goals. Rather than saying that the client is **unable to perform** a given activity, such as dress her lower body independently, it is better to give the assist level needed. In that way, you are able to measure progress as the client improves. In other words, if your problem statement reads,

Client is unable to dress self Ⓘ due to ↓ AROM in Ⓑ UE.

You will not be able to show any increase in function until the client is independent in dressing. If you word your problem statement to show the amount that the AROM is decreased and the current level of assistance needed,

Client needs max Ⓐ to dress self due to ½ AROM in Ⓑ UE.

then, as soon as the client is able to regain enough active range to dress with mod Ⓐ, or shows an increase in AROM, you can document progress. It may sometimes be useful to add the cause, such as,

Client needs max Ⓐ in dressing due to ½ AROM in Ⓑ UE 2° to infection of the spinal cord.

It is not mandatory to add the causative factor. Sometimes it is irrelevant or unknown. It is sometimes helpful since there may be a difference in the interventions that will be provided based on the cause.

Usually if a client is unable to perform an activity Ⓘ the assist level will be specified. However, sometimes the activity is one that the client either can or cannot do, with no assist levels in question. In that case, you can use the following format:

Client unable to _____ due to _____.
　　　　　　　　Engage in what occupational task　　　　　　　What underlying factor

For example,

Consumer is unable to sustain employment more than 2 weeks due to absence of stress management skills.

Client is unable to grasp a writing instrument for more than 3 minutes due to pain level of >5/10 with flexion of Ⓡ fingers.

Child is unable to do jumping jacks to participate in gym class due to motor planning deficits.

In this case, the child cannot do the task with any level of assistance. It is a can or can't activity. The child is not Ⓓ in jumping jacks, she just can't do them.

It is not mandatory that the above formats be used. These are useful ways of wording, but there are others. Sometimes a slightly different format is more useful:

_____ results in _____.
　　　Underlying factor　　　　　　　　What occupational deficit

For example:

Three steps leading to front door limit client's independence in entering house.

Inability to calculate results is a need for caregiver assistance in IADL tasks such as balancing checkbook.

Pain level >6 at end ranges limits ability to move through full AROM to participate in self-care.

Aggressive behavior results in limited opportunities for social participation and repeated involvement with the juvenile justice system.

> **Note:** Just as a humanitarian reminder, please write in terms of what the client needs, rather than stating that the client is a particular assist level. Our clients are much more than their assist levels. In this manual you will find the client referred to as patient, client, consumer, veteran, child, resident, or individual in various notes. All of these are commonly used and vary by facility. Please use the term that is considered most respectful in your setting.

Please say: *"Veteran needs or requires max assist..."*

rather than　*"Veteran is max assist..."*

Please say: *"Individual will dress with mod assist..."*

rather than *"Individual will be mod assist in dressing..."*

The language we use in speaking of clients reminds us that they are more than their disabilities or limitations and deserve our respect.

Examples of Functional Problem Statements

Cognition
Individual requires verbal and tactile cues 100% of the time in order to stay on task, initiate, and sequence during dressing activity.

Belief in a government conspiracy limits consumer's willingness to participate socially.

Impaired short-term memory makes client unsafe to cook or care for young children.

Communication
Veteran unable to communicate verbally 2° intubation.

Consumer needs mod verbal cues to initiate social conversation 2° low self-esteem.

Dressing
Client requires mod Ⓐ to don pants 2° 3+ upper extremity strength.

Patient requires mod verbal cues and mod physical assist with upper body dressing 2° attention span of <5 minutes.

Preference for youth-culture specific dress limits client's ability to find employment.

Endurance (Activity Tolerance)
Client tolerates < 10 minutes ADL secondary to shortness of breath.

Client unsafe in home management tasks due to inability to recognize fatigue when standing.

Feeding
Individual unable to keep food on fork due to poor motor planning.

Limited food preferences interfere with balanced nutritional intake.

As a result of increased tactile defensiveness, child is unable to eat textured foods.

Grooming/Self-Care
Patient requires mod Ⓐ in dressing and hygiene activities 2° low vision.

Veteran requires max Ⓐ in combing hair with Ⓡ UE due to pain in Ⓡ elbow.

Client unsafe and mod Ⓐ in bathing 2° poor balance and lack of adaptive equipment.

Inattention to personal hygiene interferes with consumer's ability to find employment.

Hands

Child needs mod (A) in upper body hygiene 2° pronator spasticity which limits supination of (R) forearm by 1/2 range.

Patient is unable to do carpentry work due to grip strength of 4# in (R) hand.

Mobility/Transfers

Resident needs max (A) in bed mobility secondary to decreased strength in trunk and UEs.

Client (D) in bed mobility due to severe UE and LE contractures.

Discomfort in crowds limits client's willingness to leave his house for social participation.

Pain

Pain level of >6/10 at end ranges limits ability to move through full AROM to participate in self-care.

Patient unable to grasp and hold tool with (L) hand due to pain level >5/10 with flexion of (L) index finger.

Fear of rejection limits consumer's willingness to venture into social settings.

Pediatrics

Child unable to do jumping jacks during gym class as a result of poor motor planning.

Child requires mod (A) to complete art assignment requiring the use of a ruler 2° bilateral in-coordination.

Patty does not transfer toys from one hand to the other due to inattention to the right side of the body.

Positioning

Child unable to feed self due to asymmetrical positioning in wheelchair.

Safety

Client unsafe in IADL tasks due to impaired judgment and sequencing.

Trace strength in shoulder, elbow & wrist flexors/extensors 2° (L) CVA results in need for mod (A) in showering safely.

Focused attention on auditory hallucinations makes consumer unsafe to live alone.

Frequent alcohol use impairs Jerry's ability to operate a motor vehicle safely.

Impaired short-term memory makes patient unsafe in home management tasks.

Sensation

Decreased (R) UE sensation results in mod (A) to perform self-care activities independently or safely.

Child is unable to engage in age-appropriate play activities due to sensory deficits.

Client needs adaptive equipment in order to return to carpentry work 2° to ↓ sensation in thumb and index finger.

Upper Extremity Use

< 60° AROM in Ⓡ shoulder abduction limits patient's ability to use Ⓡ UE for upper body ADL and work tasks.

Child's weak intrinsic hand muscles and incoordination result in an inability to cut circles and straight lines in class.

Mental Health

Individual's aggressive behavior results in social isolation.

Consumer needs mod assist in IADL tasks due to inattention to his environment.

Belief in a government conspiracy results in Jim being reluctant to leave his house for social participation.

Attention to the voices she is hearing interferes with Mary's ability to care for her children.

Substance Abuse

Client has been using alcohol and drugs on a regular basis for at least 1 year, resulting in inability to complete home management tasks.

Drug seeking and using behaviors limit Andy's social participation in non-drug related activities.

Consumer admits to using cocaine on a daily basis resulting in inability to hold a job.

Habit of getting drunk at all holiday celebrations limits Mr. D.'s invitations to participate socially with family and friends.

For more examples of problem statements in mental health and chemical dependency, see Chapter 11.

Note: Problem Statements in Mental Health and Substance Abuse

In mental health and substance abuse practice settings, problem statements are usually multidisciplinary, and written to be addressed by the treatment team rather than by one specific discipline. Although goals for mental health and substance abuse can be written in the format shown above, in practice they are often done as a two-part statement. For example:

Problem: Alcohol use

Behavioral Manifestations: Bill admits to drinking 8 oz. of liquor and 7 to 8 beers nightly, resulting in failing grades and involvement with the law due to fighting with fists and weapons.

WORKSHEET 3-2

Writing Functional Problem Statements

Please use the following problems to write functional problem statements. Make them specific enough to:

- Show the area of occupation that is at risk.
- Show the underlying factors that are not WFL.
- Serve as a baseline against which to measure progress.

You may use any of the three formats given for writing your problem statements.

1. The client has acquired an injury to his brain. As a result, he is not able to pay attention to task for very long at a time, and is having trouble completing his morning routine. Usually he can pay attention to what he is doing for about 2 minutes, and needs to be redirected back to the task after that.

2. The child is having trouble in school because she has difficulty staying within the lines when she is writing. She habitually grips her pencil in a gross grasp, although with help (someone's hand placed over hers) she can hold it with her thumb and two fingers.

3. The resident is not very cognitively aware. About 40% of the time she has trouble figuring out what to do first if she has to complete a self-care task, and she doesn't remember what she has just been told.

4. Mr. J. has recently sustained a Ⓡ CVA. His Ⓛ upper extremity is flaccid and he forgets that it is there. He needs physical and verbal help with ADL tasks about 60% of the time.

5. The consumer has had trouble finding a job. His appearance is unkempt and he has a strong body odor, neither of which appear troubling to him.

6. The client is unable to transfer safely w/c ↔ toilet without someone to remind him that he needs to follow his total hip precautions.

Chapter 4
WRITING FUNCTIONAL AND MEASURABLE GOALS AND OBJECTIVES

Goals and objectives used in a treatment plan must be written in functional, measurable, observable, action-oriented terms. They must also be realistic for the client and able to be achieved in a reasonable amount of time. Goals are formulated from the problem list you have compiled in collaboration with the client. For successful intervention, it is critical that you work on goals that are important to the client. Do not assume that because your client is not very alert or able to communicate that he does not know what he wants (Kannenberg & Greene, 2003).

Occupational therapy goals must focus on functional gains. The client factors or biomechanical gains that underlie such progress are much less important to a third party payer than what the client can actually do, even though the gains in underlying factors may be essential to achieving the functional outcome.

As a profession, we are increasingly being asked to show evidence that our intervention strategies work and that they are cost effective (Mandich, Miller, & Law, 2002). There is an emphasis on outcomes that move beyond the physical impairments to increase the client's ability to function within the environment and to improve quality of life. This move to evidence-based practice reminds us of how important it is to establish outcome measures that demonstrate functional improvements and ability to participate in meaningful occupation.

Goals

Goals in an intervention plan are also called **long-term goals** (LTG) or outcomes. These are usually discharge goals—what the client hopes to accomplish by the time of discharge. For each problem you have identified, you will have at least one long-term goal, and often more than one.

Objectives

Objectives are also called **short-term goals** (STG). These are the daily goals that are met while progressing toward the discharge goals. For example, if your long-term goal is:

In order to perform job without injury, client will be able to move 35# objects needed for work from table to counter without ↑ in pain by 12/18/05.

then one of your short-term goals might be:

In order to perform job tasks, client will be able to lift 10# objects needed for work without increase in pain by 12/5/05.

If your long-term goal is:

In order to return to independent living situation, client will transfer independently and safely bed ↔ wheelchair standing pivot while wearing an orthotic foot support within 2 weeks.

then one of your short-term goals might be:

In order to be independent and safe in standing pivot transfers required for returning home, client will reach for bed or wheelchair before sitting with no verbal cues within 1 week.

You may have several short-term goals (objectives) for each long-term goal. For example, suppose you are treating Mr. Hawkins, a 45-year-old executive who sustained a (R) CVA a few days ago and has (L) side hemiplegia. On evaluation you find that he is oriented X4, verbal, intelligent, able to learn, and has a supportive wife. After talking with him about what he would like to achieve in occupational therapy, you and he decide upon a goal of independent upper body dressing. You believe that this is a realistic goal, provided that he receives skilled instruction and the correct adaptive equipment.

You set a series of objectives:

1.   In order to begin dressing activities, client will be able to maintain dynamic sitting balance at edge of bed for >5 minutes while reaching for clothing at arms' length by the end of the 3rd treatment session.
2.   By the 6th treatment session, client will be able to tolerate > 10 minutes of dressing sitting edge of bed.
3.   After skilled instruction, client will be able to don shirt sitting EOB using the over-the-head method by 7/10/05.
4.   After skilled instruction, client will be able to button shirt using a buttonhook by 7/12/05.
5.   While sitting on edge of bed, client will be independent in upper body dressing by 7/15/05.

As you can see, each of these short-term goals is measurable, observable, and client-action oriented. The first four short-term goals are steps to the ultimate long-term goal (Figure 4-1).

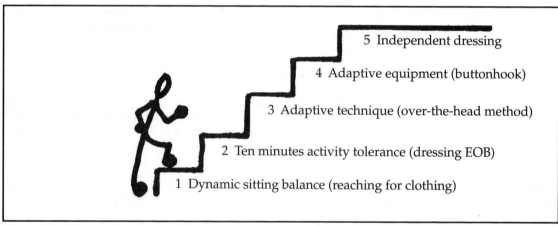

Figure 4-1. Steps to the ultimate LTG.

An intervention plan is always a work in progress. Unexpected events and conditions can impact the progress your client will be able to make toward his or her goals. If you find a goal unrealistic, you are obligated to change it. It is not useful to continue with a plan that is not working.

For example, suppose that your client, Mr. Hawkins, begins to have some return in his involved (L) upper extremity. You now know that he may be able to dress his upper body without adaptive techniques or equipment, and he wants very much to do that. After we discuss the format for writing goals, you might write a new set of short-term goals for Mr. Hawkins.

Goal Writing: The FEAST Method

F – Function	For what occupational gain?
E – Expectation	The client will
A – Action	Do what?
S – Specific Condition	Under what conditions?
T – Timeline	By when?

In order to write goals and objectives in a way that can be measured, the elements to be included are very specific. The FEAST format is useful as you are learning to write, although the order may need to be changed slightly in order for your sentence to make sense. As long as all the required elements are present, you can begin with any of the elements—the expectation, the conditions, the timeline, or the function.

Now let's look at each category a little more closely:

F (Function)

This is the specific area of occupation to which this goal pertains, if it is not imbedded in the goal. For example "in order to return to work as a carpenter" or "in order to be able to be bathed by his caretakers" or "in order to be able to write his name at school." For example,

> *In order to begin writing his name at school, the student will demonstrate ability to hold a crayon using tripod pinch by 10/19/05.*

The function may go after the action if you prefer. For example,

> *The student will be able to hold a crayon using tripod pinch in order to learn to write his name at school by 10/19/05.*

Often the function is the same as the action.

> *The client will perform a three-step cooking process at wheelchair level by 3/16/05.*

In this case the function (cooking) is inherent in the goal and does not need to be restated.

Function is the ability to engage in occupation, and is the core of occupational therapy practice. It is the **first** thing you think of in writing goals, and should be the essential focus of the goal statement.

E (Expectation)

In writing treatment goals, the **client** is the key player. You set the expectation:

> *The client will . . .*

Note: These are the client's goals. The goal statement is not the place to tell what the therapist will do. That goes later, under intervention strategies.

A (Action)

An action verb is inserted here, such as perform, demonstrate, identify, cook, don, comb, unfasten, or complete, followed by the skill to be performed. For example,

> *The client will **perform a three-step cooking process.***

In this case, the function is contained in the action statement, and does not need to be added.

S (Specific Condition)

This is the level of assistance expected and/or the conditions under which the client is expected to be able to perform the desired action. For example: "...after set up"; ". . .by using a dressing stick"; ". . .at wheelchair level"; or ". . .after skilled instruction."

> *The client will perform a three step cooking process **at wheelchair level**...*

The conditions make your goal more specific. Usually it is helpful to put the condition *after* the skill rather than before it, but sometimes you may want to start with the condition. For example,

> **After skilled instruction** *the client will be able to perform a three-step cooking process...*

Below are some examples of goals in which the conditions have been highlighted for emphasis. One of the most common mistakes in goal writing is omission of the conditions under which the activity is expected to be performed.

> *In order to dress himself with minimum assistance, client will button at least three buttons on his shirt* **using a buttonhook** *by 10/1/05.*

> *In order to be able to begin skilled instruction in dressing by 11/30/05, client will maintain static sitting balance* Ⓘ **on side of bed** *for 3 minutes.*

> *After skilled instruction, client will demonstrate proper use of sock-aid to don socks* Ⓘ *safely* **while seated in w/c** *by end of 6ᵗʰ treatment session.*

> *In order to don pants* **completely over hips** *client will demonstrate ability to transfer sit → stand* Ⓘ *within 1 week.*

T (Timeline)

This is the time frame within which the goal is expected to be accomplished. For example "...by discharge on 3/16/05" or "...by the end of the next treatment session" or "...within 2 weeks".

> **The client will perform a three-step cooking process at wheelchair level by 3/16/05.**

Medical Necessity

As occupational therapists, we view a client holistically, considering the whole person with his needs, interests, problems, strengths, and priorities rather than focusing in on a "faulty part" of the mechanism. We know that leisure is an important part of the total picture. When this is the client's priority, we might be inclined to write goals focusing on leisure skills and interests. For example,

Problem:
> *Client unable to play softball due to ↓ AROM and ↑ pain in* Ⓛ *wrist.*

LTG:
> *In order to resume his role as a team member of a softball team, client will demonstrate AROM of the* Ⓛ *wrist WFL without pain within 6 weeks.*

STG:
> *In order to prepare for resuming his role as a softball team member, client will demonstrate wrist stabilization for 1 minute while holding a 1# ball within 2 weeks.*

As knowledgeable health care professionals, we also know that both Medicare and managed care organizations are very frugal with our health care dollars and approve expenditures only for medical necessity. Since even adaptive equipment such as a raised toilet seat is not always considered medically necessary, treatment focused on the client's leisure goals is likely to be denied under our current reimbursement system. In consideration of the client's total needs and the reimbursement considerations, we may address in the intervention plan some of the underlying factors that enable the client to perform a variety of functional tasks. Documentation would include interventions that provide the client with skills for self-care and work activities and also leisure activities so important to the quality of life.

In the example above, we might suspect that the client is having difficulty with household or work tasks requiring Ⓑ upper body use as well as having trouble playing ball. It would work much better to choose IADL tasks which also require ↑ AROM and the ability to hold a 1# object for 1 minute as goals, knowing that improving these client factors and performance skills would also give the client an increased ability to pursue his leisure interests.

In the next worksheet, you will have an opportunity to rewrite leisure goals for a client so that they focus on performance skills and patterns. In this way, a payer will be able to see the medical necessity of the service being provided.

WORKSHEET 4-1
Choosing Goals for Health Necessity

Problem:
  Client unable to perform sewing due to 2+ strength in Ⓡ *hand musculature.*

LTG:
  Client will be able to perform embroidery Ⓘ *for 20 minutes within 5 months.*

STG:
  In order to ↑ performance of embroidery, client will be able to use needle continuously for 5 minutes by 11/6/05.

What other problems might this woman have due to decreased strength in her Ⓡ **hand?**

What long-term goal might you use that would show medical necessity for increasing Ⓡ **UE strength?**

What short-term goal might be used as a step to that LTG?

Stringent requirements necessitate documentation that demonstrates a clear indication of the need for skilled occupational therapy. Once a client reaches the level of minimal assistance, the changes become more subtle, and may lead to denial of payment unless the necessity of skilled occupational therapy is specified. For example, dressing with minimal assist does not necessarily indicate a need for skilled occupational therapy. However "minimal assistance with verbal instruction for over-the-head method of donning of shirt" justifies skilled occupational therapy.

Educational Goals

Therapists working in the public schools use a slightly different terminology. In education, goals for 1 school year are called **objectives**. Educational goals are not measured by time, e.g., *by 5/7/05* or *within 3 weeks*. Since the IEP is rewritten annually, the time frame for educational goals is assumed to be annual. Children sometimes exhibit a new behavior inconsistently before it is really established. Therefore, measurement used for children is more likely to reflect whether or not the behavior is established. For example,

> *Kevin will hold pencil in a tripod grasp in 3/3 opportunities.*

> *Johnny will demonstrate improved tolerance to tactile media as evidenced by self-initiation during art activities in 5/5 teacher reports.*

Goals for children in the public schools must be set in terms of a behavior that is needed in the classroom. While you may be working on sensory integration as a treatment goal, such as maintaining prone extension posture over a therapy ball, it must be written in language that relates to performance in the classroom setting.

> *Bobby will maintain upright sitting posture during writing time without verbal reminders in 3/3 observations.*

> **DO NOT** use participation in treatment as a goal. For example,
>
> *Client will do 20 reps of shoulder ladder with 1# wt. in order to ↑ endurance to become more ① in ADLs.*
>
> In a goal such as this, specify the amount of ↑ endurance you hope or expect to see. For example,
>
> *Client will be able to participate in cooking task > 5 minutes without rest breaks.*

Examples of Goal Statements

Basic Activities of Daily Living

Dressing
> *Child will be able to don coat using over-the-head method ① within 1 month.*

> *In order to button shirt ①, patient will demonstrate Ⓡ thumb MP flexion of no less than 50° within 2 weeks.*

Hygiene

Patient will complete grooming and hygiene activities with a reported pain level of <3/10 within 3 tx. sessions.

Client will brush teeth, comb hair, and shave with less than 3 verbal cues to redirect attention to task within 1 week.

Eating/Feeding

Resident will feed self a meal with correct use of adaptive equipment (lipped plate, rocker knife, and built-up angled utensils) after set up with no more than 10 verbal cues within 30 days.

Consumer will choose at least 2 food items other than pizza that he is willing to include in his diet within 1 week.

Functional Mobility

In order to return to living at home, patient will be able to propel w/c up ramp and through all doors with min Ⓐ within 2 weeks.

In order to shop Ⓘ, consumer will explain the bus schedule including which stops she commonly uses within 2 weeks.

Instrumental Activities of Daily Living

In order to return to living unassisted, patient will demonstrate an ability to locate phone numbers of emergency services in the telephone directory without physical or verbal cues after the 3rd treatment session.

In order to grocery shop Ⓘ, client will locate proper aisle within 5 minutes of entering grocery store next treatment session.

Education

In order to complete writing activities, Steve will be able to maintain upright posture at desk for >5 minutes without verbal cues within 6 weeks.

In order to increase fine motor skills needed for school, child will demonstrate Ⓘ pincer pinch pattern 5/5 times during classroom activities.

Work

Consumer will Ⓘ request a job application from a restaurant within 1 week.

In order to return to carpentry work, patient will demonstrate Ⓡ UE grip strength >40# within 4 weeks.

Play

In order to engage in developmental play activities, child will sit unsupported for 3 minutes within 2 months.

Bobby will use Ⓛ UE as a functional assist 5/5 opportunities during spontaneous play within 2 months.

Leisure

Client will identify at least 3 leisure activities that are not associated with drinking by 9/8/05.

Within 1 month, client will demonstrate sufficient coordination to manipulate toothpaste caps, buttons, and knitting needles without dropping.

Social Participation

Consumer will choose and participate in at least one social activity per week 3/3 weeks within 1 month.

With mod verbal cues, consumer will ask roommate to smoke outside the building.

WORKSHEET 4-2
Evaluating Goal Statements

Refer to your FEAST elements to determine which of the following goals has each of the necessary components to be useful in occupational therapy documentation. For each goal that you find to be incomplete or inaccurate in some way, indicate what it lacks.

1. *By the time of discharge in 2 weeks, client will be able to dress himself with min (A) for balance using a sock aid and reacher while sitting in a wheelchair.*
   __ This goal has all the necessary components to be useful.
   __ This goal lacks

2. *Client will tolerate 10 minutes of treatment daily.*
   __ This goal has all the necessary components to be useful.
   __ This goal lacks

3. *Client will demonstrate increased coping skills in order to live at home with her granddaughter within 2 weeks.*
   __ This goal has all the necessary components to be useful.
   __ This goal lacks

4. *Client will demonstrate 15 minutes of activity tolerance without rest breaks using (B) UE in order to complete ADL tasks before breakfast each morning.*
   __ This goal has all the necessary components to be useful.
   __ This goal lacks

5. *In order to be able to toilet self (I) after discharge, client will demonstrate ability to perform a sliding board transfer w/c → mat within the next week.*
   __ This goal has all the necessary components to be useful.
   __ This goal lacks

6. *OT will teach lower body dressing using a reacher, dressing stick, and sock aid within 3 tx. sessions.*
   __ This goal has all the necessary components to be useful.
   __ This goal lacks

7. *In order to return to living independently, patient will demonstrate ability to balance his checkbook.*
   __ This goal has all the necessary components to be useful.
   __ This goal lacks

WORKSHEET 4-3

Writing Realistic, Functional, Measurable Goals

Write measurable, functional, time limited, realistic goals for the scenarios below. Please remember that we set goals with the client. Assume for this practice sheet that you have already collaborated with the client regarding his/her goals.

1. Mary is not able to attend to task for more than a few minutes, which makes IADL activities difficult for her. Since she likes to cook and plans to return to cooking after discharge, you have been working with her in the kitchen. You would like to see her able to attend to task for 10 minutes by the time she is discharged next week. Write a goal to increase Mary's attention span.

F (if not included in action below)_____

(For what functional gain)

E _____

(Expectation—the client will)

A _____

(Action)

S _____

(Specific conditions)

T _____

(Time line—by when?)

2. Now write a goal for Mary to be able to follow directions so that she can read the back of a boxed meal, and eventually a recipe, when she is cooking.

F (if not included in action)_____

E _____

A _____

S _____

T _____

3. Bill is having trouble dressing himself after his stroke. You have been teaching him an over-the-head method for putting on his shirt, and have given him a buttonhook to use. Write a dressing goal for Bill.

F (if not included in action)_____

E _____

A _____

S _____

T _____

4. Susan is very weak, and wants to be able to go back to work as a receptionist. She also wants to be able to care for her 4-month-old child. Write a goal to increase her activity tolerance. Discharge is ~2 weeks away.

F (if not included in action)_____

E _____

A _____

S _____

T _____

5. Sam wants to live independently in the community, but lacks basic money management skills. Write a goal for Sam to improve his money management skills.

F (if not included in action)_____

E _____

A _____

S _____

T_____

6. Audrey has become increasingly more depressed over the past several weeks, and was admitted after a suicide attempt. You estimate that you will have her in groups for 1 week. You would like to see her mood change in that week. Write a goal that will indicate an improved mood.

F (if not included in action)_____

E _____

A _____

S _____

T _____

Chapter 5
WRITING THE "S"—SUBJECTIVE

The first section of the SOAP note contains **subjective** information obtained from the client, giving his perspective on his condition or treatment. Subjective data is information that cannot be verified or measured during the treatment session. In this section, the therapist records the client's report of limitations, concerns, and problems, as well as what the client said that was relevant to treatment, such as significant complaints of pain, fatigue, or expressions of feelings, attitudes, concerns, goals, and plans. When direct quotes are used in the subjective section of the SOAP note, it is understood that the statement comes from the individual receiving the therapy, unless otherwise stated.

The information obtained from the client will be of greater significance and relevance to the rest of your note if it is specific rather than general in nature. For instance, if the client tells you, "My shoulder hurts," you may question him further, asking him "Where does it hurt?" or "When does it hurt?", so your note can communicate more detailed information on his condition. His description might be written as: *Client states his* Ⓡ *shoulder hurts when he tries to put his shirt on.* You may use a quote or summarize what the client said.

Examples of "S" Statements

"I don't need therapy."

Resident reports pain in Ⓡ *shoulder when reaching up to comb hair.*

Patient asked for help when it was needed during dressing.

Client reports, "I keep blowing up at home, and yelling at everyone, and I don't know what to do about it."

"I can't wash the dishes or zip my coat."

Veteran reports that his fingers "look kind of dead."

Patient reported he needed to go to meet someone and get to work when the session began. When asked questions such as "Can you hear me?" he often responded, "I need to go."

Resident reports he feels "pretty good" now and his goal is to "get back as natural" as he can.

Consumer reports being fearful of leaving her home.

Client reports that his doctor has ordered "some home care for a few days to work on transfers."

Client reported that her shoulders feel better after taping. "My short-term goal is to be able to write, and my long-term goal is to return to work."

Martha called the emergency line last night to report a burning sensation in her "gut" which made her afraid she was going to die. Today she reports that she has been worrying about dying and has not showered since the day before yesterday.

Resident reports being able to bathe and dress self (I), but does not open dresser drawers and closet doors due to a fall from opening a dresser drawer which resulted in a hip fracture. She was able to tell the correct day and month when asked.

Patient commented that she used to use her (L) hand to hold a cup but now is unable to do so. Patient also complained of soreness in (L) shoulder and inquired about finding a student to assist her at home upon discharge.

Client stated that she has experienced several episodes of bladder incontinence when trying to make it to the bathroom.

Consumer contributed to ~25% of the group discussion, reporting that the hardest feelings for her to deal with are worry and fear about her physical problems, which might go undetected. She reports being unable to function at home (cannot cook, keep house, or do laundry) when she is "sick with depression," but wants to do these things again. Consumer reports that exercise, prayer, and volunteer work are her primary coping strategies, and that she would like to learn more about relaxation techniques.

In an evaluation, the "S" may contain all or part of the occupational profile:

Client reports that she was admitted after a fall that resulted in confusion and left-sided weakness. Prior to admission, she was living alone in a one story home and was (I) in all activities of daily living. She reports that she is a retired librarian, widowed 10 years ago. She says she values her independence and fully intends to return to her own home. She reports that her activities are primarily sedentary, including sewing, reading, and playing cards with friends. She says her daughter lives two blocks away and provides transportation when needed.

The client talked about his current symptoms and the events leading up to his hospitalization. He reports losing his job with United Construction after not reporting for work for 2 weeks due to depression, having an argument with his wife, and taking an overdose. He says that he has always "worked construction" and does not know how to do anything else. He reports concern that his former employer will not give him "a decent reference." He says he really has no leisure interests except going out "drinking with the guys after work" and sometimes going hunting in the fall.

Sometimes the client is not able to speak or does not make any relevant comments. In such cases, include that information in the "S" section.

For example:

Client unable to communicate due to aphasia.

Client did not speak without cueing.

Patient communicated using her message board that she wanted to be able to take care of herself.

Resident does not clearly verbalize during treatment, but smiles and nods appropriately when asked questions.

Occasionally you will include information that the family provided about the client if this is pertinent to the note or client's progress. When treating infants and very young children, you may report what the parent says. Except for infants and people who are not able to communicate, the "S" section is usually reserved for the client's view.

Common Errors

Not Using Communication Time With the Client Effectively

The most common error that new therapists make in gathering subjective information is in failing to make good use of communication with the client during treatment sessions. Instead of using the time in therapy to talk socially, a good therapist will use the time to listen effectively and to ask questions that will provide pertinent information about the client's attitudes and concerns; this information can be used to ensure effective treatment as well as appropriate documentation. Instead of talking to your client about the weather or Monday Night Football, why not ask him how he thinks he is doing in therapy or what his feelings are related to his upcoming discharge placement? As therapists gain experience, they begin to use the treatment session to provide relevant data regarding such things as occupational history, functional status, prior level of functioning, motivation, priorities, and family support.

Effective communication and interviewing during treatment sessions can seem just like a conversation on the surface. But, as a skilled therapist, you are directing the conversation to topics that are meaningful to client care rather than allowing it to remain superficial. Use this opportunity to expand your occupational profile and gather data that are vital to providing the very best occupational therapy possible. In having a conversation with your client, guide the discussion to your client's history, problems, needs, strengths, support systems, living situation, and goals for treatment. Without knowing these things from your client's point of view, you will have difficulty planning effective treatment. When a therapist does not listen effectively during treatment, the "S" may read:

Client talked about grandchildren visiting.
-or-
Patient said "ouch" when elbow was ranged beyond 45°.

While these statements are within the scope of the "S," they are not particularly helpful pieces of information to spend time and space reporting.

Not Writing Concise, Coherent Statements

The second most common error made by new therapists in writing the subjective section of the note is that of simply listing any remarks the client makes about his condition.

For example, during one treatment session the client said the following:

"I can't feel anything with my hands."

"I'm wobbly as all get out today."

Client expressed dizziness after bending down to touch the floor while in a seated position.

Client acknowledged improvement in his sitting balance in comparison to the previous week.

Many of these statements have to do with stability, balance, and safety. While the quotations are a very objective way of reporting data, and all the statements are relevant to the intervention session, it is more effective to summarize the client's remarks in a concise and coherent manner, instead of listing each of these statements separately in the "S" section of the note. For example:

> *Client expressed lack of sensation in both hands and dizziness in sitting position with dynamic movement (a "wobbly" sensation). He also acknowledged improvement in sitting balance since last week.*
>
> -or-
>
> *Client acknowledged improved sitting balance compared to previous week. However, he experienced dizziness after bending down while sitting, and reported feeling "wobbly." Client also reported inability to feel anything with his hands.*

In the next exercise you will have the opportunity to combine a client's statements into a coherent and concise "S" statement.

WORKSHEET 5-1
Writing Concise, Coherent Statements

Ms. P. is recovering from a total hip replacement. During a treatment session, she makes the following statements.

I used that dressing stick and sock aid like you showed me to get dressed without bending down this morning.

My hip doesn't hurt when I stand up or sit down, especially with that new toilet seat you got for me.

It's getting easier for me to get dressed now.

My daughter said they delivered all that bathroom equipment to her house yesterday.

Using these statements, write your own concise and organized version for the "S" portion of the SOAP note.

S:

WORKSHEET 5-2

Choosing a Subjective Statement

An occupational therapist wrote the following observation after treating Mrs. W., a 62-year-old woman who had a stroke 3 weeks ago:

O: Client seen in rehab clinic for 30 minutes for UE activities to ↑ AROM in Ⓡ shoulder, activity tolerance, UE strength, and dynamic standing balance, in order to ↑ independence in ADL tasks.

ADL*: Client seen in room for instruction in safety techniques and adaptive equipment use in toileting. Client needs bilateral grab bars in bathroom to sit → stand safely. Client attempted to stand while pulling on walker and one grab bar. Client was instructed on safety issues and the use of bilateral grab bars, which she reported understanding.*

Performance skills*: Client sit ↔ stand CGA for balance. Client worked on activity tolerance, dynamic standing balance, and ↑ AROM in Ⓡ shoulder by moving canned goods from counter to cupboard for 5 minutes before needing a 2-minute sitting rest. After resting, she participated in activities to ↑ dynamic standing balance by pouring liquid from a pitcher while standing CGA for balance. After a 1-minute rest, client continued activities to ↑ dynamic standing balance and safety in ADL activities by pushing wheeled walker while picking up objects from floor c̄ a reacher.*

Client factors*: AROM in right shoulder abduction < 90°. PROM Ⓡ shoulder abduction WNL.*

The treatment session included all of the following. Which would be best to use as the subjective section of the SOAP note?

1. Client was cooperative and engaged in social conversation throughout the treatment session.

2. Client remarked that her grandson will be coming to visit later in the week, and that she will be very glad to see him.

3. Client reports that she feels "pretty good" today.

4. Client says she has difficulty moving Ⓡ UE, although she does not know why it will not move. She reports, "It really doesn't hurt. It's just tight."

5. Nursing staff report client is unsafe to toilet independently.

From Borcherding S. *Documentation Manual for Writing SOAP Notes in Occupational Therapy, Second Edition.*
© 2005 SLACK Incorporated

Chapter 6
WRITING THE "O"—OBJECTIVE

The second section of the note is **objective** where you will record all measurable, quantifiable, and observable data obtained during the treatment session. In this section, you will present a picture of the intervention session you have provided. Once you start looking at things with your professional eyes, they can look quite different. Instead of seeing a child playing with a toy, now you begin to note the child's asymmetrical posture, his bilateral hand use, ability to cross midline, and his pinch and grasp patterns. The trick in writing the "O" is in knowing what kind of material to include and what to omit. At first your "O" may tend to be longer than that of an experienced therapist, but with time you will learn to write notes that are both complete and concise.

Organization of the "O"

There are different ways that are acceptable in organizing the information in your observation. You may choose to present the information chronologically, discussing each treatment event in the order it occurred during that treatment session.

> *Client attended anger management group for 45 minutes today with verbal prompting by nursing staff and security aides. He displayed his displeasure at being asked to attend the group by using profanity. During the group, client related 2 instances in which individuals on the unit consistently bother him, and discussed the way he usually handles this situation. Peer feedback was given on other possible ways he might handle the same situation.*

Alternately, you may choose to organize your information into categories. When categorizing your information, choose the categories that make sense for your note. For example, suppose that today you saw June W. in the kitchen for a cooking session in preparation for discharge. She plans to cook when she returns home, but you are not certain of her safety or her ability to perform all steps of the activities from her chair. You wonder if her strength, activity tolerance, ability to use her involved hand and arm are sufficient for cooking, and you also want to assess her judgment and ability to problem solve. You choose the following categories:

- Functional mobility
- UE range and strength
- Hand function and strength
- Activity tolerance
- Cognition

Your note might look like this:
> *O: Client seen for 1 hour in clinic kitchen for skilled instruction in compensatory techniques for cooking.*
> ***Functional mobility****: Client maneuvered throughout kitchen in w/c with verbal cues to place w/c in appropriate position for reaching objects in kitchen. Client min Ⓐ in stabilizing items while transporting items in lap and maneuvering w/c simultaneously.*
> ***UE ROM and strength****: WFL for reaching items in drawers, opening oven door, and putting dishes in the sink Ⓘ. UE strength adequate for opening refrigerator door and stirring batter Ⓘ. Client requires min Ⓐ in opening Tupperware container.*
> ***Hand function and strength****: Adequate for unscrewing lids, cracking egg, and opening muffin box Ⓘ. Client able to use necessary tools for carrying out task Ⓘ. Client able to set oven dial and put muffins in oven Ⓘ.*

> ***Activity tolerance****: Client took 3-minute break after ~20 minutes of activity* $\textcircled{I}$*.*
> ***Cognition****: Client able to respond to verbal instructions and questions with correct response 3/3 times. Client said she did not think it would be safe for her to take the muffins out of the oven. Client able to problem-solve* $\textcircled{I}$ *about repositioning her w/c 75% of tx. time.*

There is no list of "correct" categories. If the client has no deficits in a particular area, it is not necessary to include that category in the note. In choosing categories, you could use the categories in the *Framework* (AOTA, 2002a). These categories are useful in any practice setting.
- Performance skills
- Performance patterns
- Context
- Activity demands
- Client factors

Sometimes, however, the *Framework* categories may be too broad for your purposes. You might choose categories that are more specific to your client and your practice setting. You may want to consider some of the following:
- Basic ADL Task Performance: Note how each of the performance skills and client factors observed impact completion of ADL tasks. Include assist levels and set-up needed, any adaptive equipment or technique used. Also include type of cueing and response, family education, positioning, and client's response to the treatment provided.
- Posture and balance: Note whether balance was static or dynamic. Consider whether the client leans in one direction, has rotated posture, even or uneven weight distribution. Notice position of the head and symmetry. Note what cues or feedback were needed to maintain or restore balance.
- Coordination: Include hand dominance, type of prehension used, ability to grasp and maintain grasp without dropping, reach and purposeful release, object manipulation, gross vs. fine motor ability.
- Swelling or edema: Give girth or volumetric measurements if possible, pitting or non-pitting, including levels if pitting.
- Movement patterns in affected upper extremity: Note tone, tremors, synergy pattern, facilitation required, stabilization, body movement.
- Ability to follow instructions: Note type and amount of instruction required, such as physical, verbal or visual cuing, ability to follow one-, two-, or three-step directions.
- Cognitive status: Report on initiation of task, verbal responses, approach to the task, ability to stay on task, sequencing, oriented X 4 (identifying time, place, person, and situation), requirements for cuing, number of steps successfully completed in task, judgment (recognition of impairments, impulsivity), ability to respond to written or verbal directions.
- Neurological factors: Note perseveration (motor, speech), sensory losses (specific), motor deficit, praxis, damage to innervation (spasticity, flaccidity, rigidity, synergy), unilateral neglect, bilateral integration, tremors.
- Functional mobility: Note the kind of assistance needed for the client to reposition him- or herself in bed, walk, propel his or her wheelchair, drive, or use public transportation (equipment, adapted technique, stand-by assistance, verbal cues).
- Psychosocial factors: Note client's overall mood, affect, and ability to engage with others. Also note family support, response to changes in body image, ability to make realistic discharge decisions for self.

Additional Categories for Mental Health or Behavioral Medicine

- Social interaction: Note awareness of others in the group, length of conversations, initiation of conversation, interaction with peers or leader in a group setting.
- Judgment and problem solving: Include any impulsivity, safety awareness, ability to identify and correct errors.
- Behavior: Report on agitation, lethargy, affect, compulsivity, anxiety, demanding behavior.
- Appearance: Note grooming, hygiene, choice of appropriate attire.
- Work Skills: Include promptness, concentration, attention span, ability to follow direction, organization of task, including preparation and clean up (Mason, personal communication, 2001).

Three Steps to Writing Good Observations

Step 1: Begin With a Statement About the Setting and Purpose of the Activity

If you are working directly on **occupation-based tasks**, use the following format for your opening:

Client seen for _____ minutes _____ for _____.
　　　　　　　　　　　　　　(In what setting)　　　　　　(Purpose of the treatment session)

In Chapter 1, you learned that some practice settings bill for OT services using CPT codes that are based on the number of minutes of each specific service the client received. Your documentation is the basis for answering any questions regarding the amount of OT the patient received. Facilities that do not charge for OT by the number of minutes may not require that you document the length of time a client was seen.

If the session is centered on improving **client factors** such as strengthening, range of motion, activity tolerance, or dynamic balance, then add a reference to the **relevant area of occupation** in the opening sentence:

Client seen for _____ minutes _____ for _____
　　　　　　　　　　　　　　(In what setting)　　　　　　(Purpose of the treatment session)
for _____.
　　(For what expected functional gain)

For example:

Pt. seen for 45 minutes in OT clinic to address ⓛ side neglect and impaired motor planning in self-care activities.

Client seen in dayroom on unit for instruction in anger management techniques needed to maintain relationships and sustain employment.

Child seen for 45 minutes in clinic to increase selective attention and fine motor manipulation as a prerequisite to enhanced play and BADL tasks.

Client seen for 60 minutes in room to provide skilled instruction in energy conservation in IADL activities and for explanation of client education materials on energy conservation.

Joe participated in role-play activity for 30 minutes in assertion group in order to explore alternative ways to get his social needs met.

Client seen for 25 minutes in outpatient clinic to increase functional movements and prehension patterns of Ⓛ hand in order to prepare for return to work.

Child seen for ½ hour in therapy room to ↑ strength and tone needed to improve handwriting in school.

Resident seen for 20 minutes in room at sink for instruction on adaptive strategies for grooming Ⓘ.

Student seen in sensory integration playroom to address sensory defensiveness in classroom activities.

Showing Your Skill

It is important to show the need for your skill as an OT in the very first sentence of your "O." For example, instead of saying *"Client seen for 45 minutes bedside for ADL training,"* you might say:

Client seen for 45 minutes bedside for instruction in compensatory dressing techniques.

Resident seen for 45 minutes bedside for instruction in use of adaptive equipment to increase safety in ADL tasks.

Veteran seen for 45 minutes bedside to facilitate attention to Ⓛ side during self-care activities.

Step 2: Follow the Opening Sentence With a Summary of What You Observed

After you have established the setting and purpose, you will discuss the intervention you have just completed, either in chronological order or in categories. Some notes work best when reported chronologically, and others work better in categories.

Julie is a 27-year-old mother of two children ages 2 and 4. She is employed in a manufacturing job that involves lifting 30-pound boxes. She is currently unable to work due to back pain from a herniated disc in her lumbar area. She complains of pain when doing her housework, and tells you that she wants to be able to perform IADL and work tasks without pain. As you do her occupational profile, you ask her to demonstrate some IADL and work tasks. As you watch her take items from the refrigerator, wash the dishes, sweep and vacuum the floor, and lift a box from the floor to a chair, you find that her body mechanics are poor and that she would benefit from client education. If you reported on your session using chronological order, you might say:

O: Client seen for 30 minutes in OT clinic for evaluation of low back pain and instruction in proper body mechanics. Client sits asymmetrically with weight shifted to her Ⓛ hip. Client demonstrated the way she usually removes items from the refrigerator, washes dishes, cleans the floors, and lifts. She was then instructed in proper body mechanics for completing these tasks, using a golfer's lift, squats, stepping toward the item she wishes to retrieve, facing the load and keeping it close to her body. Client demonstrated these techniques correctly and was given educational materials to remind her of correct positioning.

If you wanted to put the same information into categories, you might say:

> Client seen for 30 minutes in OT clinic for evaluation of low back pain and instruction in proper body mechanics.
>
> **Bending and lifting**: Client demonstrated her usual way of moving items from low surfaces to higher ones, demonstrating incorrect body mechanics in back extension and bending at the waist. After instruction in using golfer's lift or squat, client demonstrated ability to use these techniques correctly in lifting and work activities after 2 attempts.
>
> **Transporting**: Client exhibited torque in the spine in transporting items such as dishes. After instruction in sidestepping, facing the load and keeping it close to the body, client demonstrated proper use of these techniques with less reported pain.
>
> **Reaching**: IADL tasks such as sweeping and vacuuming also habitually performed with rotation and overextension of the back. After instruction and demonstration of moving the body rather than overextending the arms, and keeping the load close to the body, client demonstrated correct body mechanics in performing reaching tasks with decreased pain.
>
> **Client education**: Client given educational materials to remind her of correct positioning for task and reported that she understood what to do.

In this case, the chronological note works better because there is some repetition in the categorized version, and the categorized version is also longer. However, some notes are better if they are divided into sections. Categories help an inexperienced therapist to focus on the performance skills the client is demonstrating rather than the media that is being used to facilitate these skills. In the next exercise, you will see a chronological note that would work better in categories.

WORKSHEET 6-1

Using Categories

Consider the following chronological observation:

Child seen for 60 minutes in daycare setting to work on reach/grasp/release and feeding skills. With min Ⓐ for facilitation of movement at elbow, child demonstrated ability to use Ⓛ UE to reach, grasp, and release 5 objects with 1 – 2 verbal cues per object and restriction of Ⓡ UE movement. Child was able to feed self Ⓘ with ~50% spillage, but demonstrated significant limitations in chewing action p̄ ~3 rotary chews & swallowing ~90% of food without chewing. Child required verbal cues throughout session to maintain attention to task. Child wore soft spica thumb splint for entire tx. session.

How would you divide this information into categories to make it easier to read? Choose 3 to 4 categories and redistribute the information above into the categories you have chosen.

Step 3: Be Professional, Concise, and Specific

The "O" section does not need to be written in complete sentences. Give complete information in the most concise form possible. Some details *must* be included. For example, ROM must be specified as active, passive, or assistive and must indicate the joint at which the movement occurred. UE or LE must indicate which UE or LE. Level of assistance must be specified if assistance was given. Below are some examples of wording changes that make your wording more professional, concise, and specific.

Rather than saying: *Resident flopped down onto bed short of breath, closed her eyes, and moaned. Resident laid in bed with min Ⓐ to position herself.*
You might say: *Client observed to be fatigued following tx. session and required min Ⓐ for positioning in bed.*

Rather than saying: *Veteran had to use a trapeze to sit up.*
You might say: *Supine → sit using trapeze.*

Rather than saying: *Client put the board in place to make a sliding board transfer.*
You might say: *Client positioned sliding board for transfer.*

When you are documenting test results, it is helpful to put them into a chart like the one below, rather than burying them in a narrative.

Sensory testing of Ⓛ hand revealed:
Hot/cold: Intact
Sharp/dull: Impaired over volar surface, intact over dorsal surface
Stereognosis: Absent

When first learning to write client observations, it is hard to decide what to include and what to leave out. At first, it is best to include too much data, rather than take a chance on omitting something important. As your observational skills become more refined, it will become second nature to include all the important data, and the "O" section of your notes will begin to be more concise. Here is a client observation written by an inexperienced therapist. In an effort to include all the necessary data, she wrote a note that was too wordy.

Client was seen in therapy room for Ⓡ UE strengthening. Client was asked to clasp hands together and raise arms above head x30. Pt was then instructed to cross her midline and touch her opposite shoulder with Ⓡ UE. Client required 6 rest periods for completion. Client completed tasks Ⓘ. Client was then introduced to weight and pulley system. Client was asked to specify how much weight she thought she could do. She responded with 5#. Client did 30 reps of the pulley system with 5# in shoulder flexion to strengthen her rotator cuff to decrease the probability of dislocating her shoulder again. After strengthening exercise client had 3 heat packs applied to shoulder to decrease pain.

A more experienced therapist might have written:

Client seen in clinic for the following Ⓡ UE strengthening exercises for rotator cuff in order to prevent further dislocation:
Ⓑ clasped hand shoulder flexion and extension x 30 repetitions
Horizontal adduction Ⓡ hand to Ⓛ shoulder x 30 repetitions
Ⓡ shoulder flexion pulleys with 5# wt. x 30 repetitions
3 hot packs used to ↓ pain after treatment

You will notice, however, that there is another problem with this note besides the fact that it is wordy. It also sounds like a physical therapy note rather than an occupational therapy note. This note needs to have functional components added, although they do not have to be in the "O." A statement from the client in the "S" about what she is unable to do with an injured rotator cuff and a statement in the "A" and/or "P" indicating functional problems/goals would suffice to make it a good occupational therapy note. Notice that being more concise means knowing what information can be omitted without compromising the quality of the observation.

It is possible to be **too** concise, omitting necessary information. For example, consider the following "O" from a community mental health center evaluation:

> **O**: Client seen in office for COPM evaluation. Client completed COPM in 45 minutes. Client responded to directive questions regarding self-care, productivity, and leisure.

This "O" does not provide much information. When additional information is added, we learn much more about the evaluation session with this client:

> **O**: Client seen in office for evaluation using the Canadian Occupational Performance Measure (COPM), which she completed in 45 minutes. She arrived 45 minutes late to the appointment, well groomed and neatly dressed. Questions regarding productivity and leisure were answered $\bar{p}$ clear enunciation and animated tone, but questions about self-care (particularly those about scar management) were declined or given short answers with sad tone and no eye contact. Client frequently touched scars on trunk during the evaluation.

It is a matter of balancing the need to be complete when writing the "O" with the need to be concise. In the next exercise you will have an opportunity to make an observation more concise, without losing any of its informational content.

WORKSHEET 6-2

Being More Concise

Now it's your turn. Revise the following note to be complete but more concise.

O: Pt seen bedside. Client ambulated ~36 inches to shower with SBA for safety. Client instructed to complete shower while sitting. Client performed shower with SBA to manage IV line. Client able to wash upper and lower body Ⓘ and dry entire body after completing shower. Client required ~20 minutes to complete shower. Client then ambulated ~36 inches to chair and sat. Client needed verbal cues to remain seated while donning underwear and pants. Client able to dress UE Ⓘ and lower body p̄ verbal cues for sitting. Client demonstrated good sitting balance, but needed SBA for standing balance. Following shower, client stated he would like to take a nap and was assisted back into bed.

Tips for Making Your Documentation Sound More Professional

Focus on Function

Make certain that occupation is integral to the note. In a treatment session devoted to self-care activities, function is obvious. However, in a session devoted to treating client factors such as strength, range and endurance; in a session where modalities are used; or in a cotreatment session, function must be addressed separately in order to justify skilled occupational therapy. For example, although the note below is an observation of a session that was devoted to performance components, it contains a statement about the functional intent of the exercises.

> **O**: *Veteran seen in room for AROM and strengthening of* Ⓛ *UE in order to regain ability to dress self. Client performed self-ranging exercises from standing and seated position with standby* Ⓐ *for balance and verbal instructions to correct errors. Client was verbally cued x5 to reach higher with* Ⓛ *UE during shoulder flexion AROM.*

Focus on the **Client's Response** to the Treatment Provided, Rather Than on What the Therapist Did

Rather than saying: *Client was reminded about hip precautions.*
You might say: *Attempting to don shoes, client required 4 verbal cues to keep hip in correct alignment.*

Rather than saying: *Client was asked orientation questions pertaining to the time of day.*
You might say: *When verbally cued to look at watch, client was unable to correctly identify time.*

Rather than saying: *Client reminded to relax.*
You might say: *UE tone moderate but relaxes with verbal cue.*

Rather than saying: *Child was asked a series of yes/no questions.*
You might say: *Child responded to yes/no questions correctly 10% of the time.*

Write From the Client's Point of View, Leaving Yourself Out

The focus of good professional writing is always on the client. Turn your sentences around so that the client is the subject of your sentence.

Rather than saying: *The OT put the client's shoes on for him.*
You might say: *Client* Ⓓ *in donning shoes.*

Rather than saying: *OT instructed the client and family in energy conservation techniques.*
You might say: *Client and family instructed in energy conservation techniques and demonstrated understanding by performing correctly.*

Be Specific About Assist Levels

When giving assist levels, be sure to note what part of the activity the client needed assistance or verbal cues to perform. For example,

Veteran doffed night garment with min Ⓐ ***to untie strings on back***.

Child needed HOH assist ***for accuracy*** *when cutting with scissors.*

*Client required verbal cues **to sit down** in order to doff hosiery.*

*Consumer able to follow bus schedule with min verbal cues **to identify correct time**.*

*Resident supine → sit in bed with min verbal cues **to roll to** Ⓡ **side**.*

*Patient stand → w/c using a standard walker with min physical Ⓐ and min verbal cues **to bring walker completely back to w/c.***

*Infant able to roll supine to prone with min tactile cues **to initiate movement**.*

*Standing pivot transfer with verbal cues **on hand placement needed for safety**.*

*Client required mod Ⓐ **to follow total hip precautions** while using long-handled sponge for washing lower legs and feet.*

In trying to be concise, sometimes inexperienced therapists make the mistake of writing an "O" that contains only a list of actions with assist levels. While this is a common error, it is **incorrect**. Simply writing a list of activities or assist levels does not show skilled OT being provided. Consider this OT's observation:

Client was seen for 1 hour in the shower room to ↑ activity tolerance and improve balance during showering, and was shown a smaller shower which simulated her home shower, in order to prepare for discharge in 1 week.
Client OX4.
Client min Ⓐ with verbal cues to sit in w/c to doff hosiery and to dry off LE.
Client spontaneously rinsed soap off hands before gripping grab bar while showering.
Client used walker going to and coming from shower room.
Client tolerated standing Ⓘ during entire shower.
Client instructed in home showering.

Now let us look at the same observation, rewritten in a more useful format:

Client was seen for 1 hour in the shower room to ↑ activity tolerance and improve balance during showering and was also shown a smaller shower which simulated her home shower, in order to prepare her for Ⓘ and safe showering after discharge in 1 week.

Mobility: *Pt walked to/from shower room Ⓘ and safely with the aid of a standard walker to provide stability in shower room while dressing/undressing.*

Cognition: *Client oriented x4.*

ADL: *Client min Ⓐ with verbal cues to sit down in order to doff hosiery and to dry LEs safely. During shower, client spontaneously rinsed soap off hands prior to gripping grab bar s̄ verbal cues. Client tolerated standing Ⓘ ~5 minutes during shower s̄ SOB. Skilled instruction provided in safe technique to use in her single shower stall and recommendations given re: grab bar placement.*

WORKSHEET 6-3

Being Specific About Assist Levels

When noting assist levels in your observation, it is not enough to note just the level of assistance required. You also need to note the part of the task that required assistance, for example:

*Resident donned pants with min Ⓐ **to pull up over hips**.*

*Client propelled w/c from room to OT clinic but required verbal cues **to avoid running into other clients**.*

Rewrite the statements below to provide a part of the task that required assistance. Since you have not seen the client, you cannot know what part really required assistance. In the usual world of professional behavior, making things up is fraud, so please keep in mind that the client you are about to imagine is just an exercise in creativity. For this exercise, you will create a client in your mind, and imagine that client doing the task. As you watch your client in your mind, notice what part of the task required assistance, and modify the sentences below accordingly.

1. *Client supine → sit with min Ⓐ; bed → w/c with mod Ⓐ.*

2. *Client required SBA in transferring w/c ↔ toilet.*

3. *Client retrieved garments from low drawers with min Ⓐ.*

4. *Brushing hair required max Ⓐ.*

5. *Client completed dressing, toileting, and hygiene with min Ⓐ.*

Deemphasize the Treatment Media

In order to improve a client's performance skills, you may use various media, such as equipment or activities that will help the client reach functional goals. However, when documenting your observations of these treatment sessions, you should deemphasize the media used, and focus instead on the performance skills. For example, an inexperienced therapist might write the following:

Client worked on placing pegs into a pegboard.

This statement may accurately describe what a casual observer would see, but as a trained professional you need to look beyond the media used and see what the client was really accomplishing. The media used here are pegs and a pegboard, but what is the performance skill? Placing pegs into a pegboard is not a skill this client needs in order to be able to care for herself, however, the performance skill she practices during this activity may well be crucial to achieving independence. Suppose the therapist had written:

Client worked on tripod pinch using pegs and a pegboard.

Notice that in this example the therapist did not simply add the performance skill to the statement *Client worked on placing pegs into a pegboard to increase tripod pinch,* but actually turned the sentence around so that the tripod pinch received the emphasis and the media was mentioned only for clarification. Suppose that the therapist had written:

Client worked on tripod pinch in order to be able to grasp objects needed for ADL tasks.

In this case, mention of the media becomes optional. She could also have written:

Client worked on tripod pinch using pegs and a pegboard in order to be able to grasp objects needed for ADL tasks.

Which of the three preceding examples do you think best describes the skilled instruction that is occurring in this treatment session? This may seem like a minor distinction, but it is important in demonstrating the need for skilled OT and the emphasis on functional outcomes in therapy.

One of the most common errors among inexperienced OTs is focusing on the media used, rather than on the performance skill that is being improved by use of the media. Consider this OT's observation:

Client was seen in rehab center for standing balance activities. Client stood to walker with min Ⓐ for balloon toss. Client used Ⓡ UE to hit balloon and was able to reach to Ⓡ and Ⓛ sides approximately 7 out of 10 tries. Activity was continued for 3 minutes. Client requested rest-break and sat for 30 seconds. Client then stood with mod Ⓐ to walker and hit balloon with Ⓛ UE for 3 minutes. Client was able to hit balloon approximately 6 out of 10 times and spontaneously switched to Ⓡ hand x2 when balloon was to her far right. Client sat for another break and to switch activities. Client stood CGA to toss beanbags with Ⓡ hand for 4 minutes. Client scored 240 points with Ⓡ hand by throwing beanbags at target. Once all beanbags were thrown, client sat for a 30-second break. Client stood with CGA for balance to toss beanbags with Ⓛ hand for 30 seconds. Client scored 150 points with Ⓛ hand by throwing beanbags at scoring target. Once all beanbags were thrown, client sat and session was ended.

When this note is rewritten to focus on the performance skills, notice the difference in professionalism in the way the note reads:

Client seen in clinic for dynamic and static standing balance activities needed for ADL and IADL tasks. Pt stood to walker with mod Ⓐ for dynamic standing balance necessary for Ⓘ showering using a balloon toss activity. Client held walker with Ⓛ hand and used Ⓡ UE to reach both Ⓡ and Ⓛ sides approximately 7/10 attempts. Client sustained activity for 3 minutes continuously and then took a 30-second rest break. Client stood to walker again with mod Ⓐ for 3 minutes of continuous activity involving weight shifting and balance required in balloon tossing. Client demonstrated ability to reach to Ⓡ and Ⓛ sides to reach for moving object approximately 6/10 times. Client demonstrated ability to spontaneously shift weight 2 times to reach object. Client took 30-second rest break before next activity. Client worked on dynamic standing balance using beanbag toss activity with target. Client stood to walker for 4 minutes of dynamic balance activity with CGA, then sat for 30-second rest. Client stood again with CGA for 3 1/2 minutes of continuous dynamic balance activity.

WORKSHEET 6-4

Deemphasizing the Treatment Media

Rewrite the following statements to emphasize the skilled OT that is actually occurring in the treatment session.

Client played catch using bilateral UEs to facilitate grasp and release pattern.

Resident put dirt into pot to halfway point, added seedling, and filled remainder of pot with dirt transferred by cup. Resident completed 3 more pots while standing 8 minutes before requiring a 5-minute rest. Resident resumed standing position to water completed pots for approximately 5 minutes.

Client painted some sungazers in crafts group to be able to see that she could do something successfully.

Make Certain That It Is Clear That You Were Not Just a Passive Observer in the Session

This will be a critical factor in reimbursement. We do not get paid to watch a client do something. To show that the skill of an occupational therapist is needed, you must be actively involved in intervention, such as evaluating or modifying the activity; otherwise it will be considered unskilled.

Rather than saying: *Client compensated for shoulder flexion by leaning forward with whole body during prehension activities.*
You might say: *Client required skilled instruction to avoid compensation at the shoulder during prehension activities.*

Rather than saying: *Client performed Home Exercise Program.*
You might say: *Home Exercise Program was observed for accurate movement patterns and updated to accommodate for progress.*

Avoid Judging the Client

Rather than saying: *Client was compliant* or Client was cooperative.
You might say: *Client demonstrated ability to follow 3-step directions and sequence WFL.*

When you are working with a client who is difficult, or whose opinions and behavior you do not agree with, it is easy to judge the client and to reflect your judgments in your observation. Below is a note written by a student who was in a difficult situation. The client "went off on" the student, refusing a sponge bath, lying about having already bathed, throwing her washcloth across the room so that the student would have to pick it up, refusing to put on her slacks, and announcing that therapy was "stupid." In spite of all this, the student wrote an observation that was nonjudgmental of the client:

Client required max encouragement to participate in therapy this AM. Client ① sit → stand & ambulating to sink. Client ① at sink c̄ simulated bathing activity using long-handled sponge. Client ① retrieved washcloth from floor using a reacher. Client ① p̄ set-up to don/ doff shoes and socks using adaptive equipment. Client retrieved gown and socks ① with a reacher. Client declined to don slacks.

Use Only Standard Abbreviations

You may use the abbreviations approved by your facility. For purposes of demonstration, a list of common abbreviations is provided in Chapter 2: The Health Record. *Do not* use any other abbreviations, even if they seem common to you. If you try to read a note containing abbreviations with which you are unfamiliar, you will understand instantly how important this is. Remember that your documentation may be read by those unfamiliar with the "shorthand" that health professionals use so freely. Suppose your chart is being read by someone who is from a different background, such as an insurance clerk or an attorney or a committee at the Lion's Club who is considering funding a piece of adaptive equipment for your client. To make your note understandable to all its readers, be judicious in applying abbreviations and keep them very standard.

Helpful Hint
Good documentation is based on accurate observation, which is based on knowing what to look for. For an experienced therapist, this becomes second nature. For a student therapist, it is helpful to review the lists in this manual and to check your observations against what your supervising therapist observed during the treatment session to be sure you are noticing the items that matter most.

Chapter 7
WRITING THE "A"—ASSESSMENT

The third section of the note is the **Assessment**, which contains the therapist's appraisal of the client's progress, functional limitations, and expected benefit from rehabilitation. In the assessment section of the note, you will interpret the meaning of the data you have presented in the "S" and the "O" sections, describing what it means in your professional judgment, and its potential impact on the client's ability to engage in meaningful occupation.

For example, during the treatment session, you may have observed that the client falls over to the left when he tries to sit unsupported at the edge of his bed. You will note both the problem (static sitting balance) and the areas of occupation in which it is a problem (transfers and basic ADL tasks). In your assessment, you might say something like:

> *Lack of static sitting balance raises safety concerns when client transfers w/c to bed or toilet, and when sitting EOB for basic hygiene and dressing tasks.*

In the assessment section of your note, you will primarily note the 3 P's: **problems, progress,** and rehab **potential**. You might also point out inconsistencies, discuss emotional components, or present some reason that something was not done as planned.

Assessing the Data

To assess the data, go sentence by sentence through the data presented in the "S" and the "O", asking yourself what it means for the client's ability to engage in meaningful occupation. Note what problems, progress, or potential for rehabilitation you see. Consider these possibilities:

Problems

Problems may include some of the following.
Safety risks:
- *Safety concerns noted when client attempted to stand without locking brakes on w/c.*
- *Poor problem solving when using the stove raises safety concerns.*
- *Client's limited coping strategies for dealing with stress raise concerns for continuing the use of self-destructive behaviors.*

Inconsistencies between client report and objective findings:
- *Although client reports anticipating no difficulty in returning to prehospitalization level of home-making activity, her left-side neglect could cause significant in-home safety risks.*
- *Although the client expresses a willingness to do ADL tasks, motor planning problems create a barrier to the task.*
- *Client verbalizes a desire to progress to the next level of responsibility, but shows ↓ behavioral control when reward incentives are unavailable.*

Factors not WFL that can be influenced by OT intervention, for example:
- *Left side weakness interferes with standing balance in tub.*
- *Left side neglect necessitates verbal cues to attend to left side during BADL tasks.*
- *Deficits in cognitive processing create a need for constant verbal cues to perform kitchen tasks safely.*

- *Continued verbal threats toward other clients indicate a need for anger management techniques.*
- *Lack of forearm supination limits Katie's ability to engage in developmental play activities.*
- *Lack of spatial orientation to identify letter shapes interferes with ability to learn to read.*
- *Continuing to isolate herself in her room rather than attending groups interferes with Molly's learning to interact with unfamiliar people and situations.*
- *Child's delayed visual motor skills for chronological age affects ability to perform kindergarten tasks.*

Progress or Indications That the Treatment Being Provided Is Effective

- *Weighted utensils decrease intention tremors by ~50% when eating.*
- *Jack is making progress toward re-entry into the community as shown by his ability to prepare for an outing, respect rules by following directions, interact socially with staff, and control his behavior ~50% of the time.*
- *Ten degree ↑ in AROM in the left elbow this week allows client to don shirt Ⓘ.*
- *Patient has shown gains since the beginning of the week by demonstrating the ability to follow 1-step commands 80% of the time during ADL tasks.*
- *Client's spontaneous participation in group discussion shows good progress in developing social interaction skills.*
- *UE strength is increasing as demonstrated by ability to pull to stand.*
- *Child's progress from 70% to 90% accuracy in shape recognition indicates good recall.*

Sometimes you will need to explain the lack of progress:
- *Patient has become more dependent in ADL tasks this week due to acute infection.*

Sometimes progress is indicated by stating that previous goals have been met or changed:
- *STG #2 (buttoning ½ inch buttons x3 on shirt) met this week.*
- *STG #4 changed to "greet other clients when entering room".*

Potential for Success in Rehabilitation

- *Ability to understand instructions and desire to return to living independently indicate good potential to return to prior living situation.*
- *Patient's ability to recall and demonstrate 3/3 hip precautions shows good potential to follow hip precautions after discharge.*
- *Patient's intact manipulative skills and fine motor coordination make him a good candidate for rehabilitation.*
- *Child's progress from 60% to 70% accuracy of reproducing shapes indicates good potential to meet goals stated in IEP.*
- *Client's ability to recognize stressors shows good potential to change self-destructive coping strategies.*
- *Participation in groups, including not interrupting, asking questions appropriately, and sharing experiences indicate good potential to benefit from psychiatric rehab program.*

Writing the Assessment

As you read carefully through the material in your "S" and your "O", it is sometimes helpful to make a quick list of things you want to discuss in the "A" section of your note. For example, consider the following "S" and "O":

S: Client stated that he gets bored during the day when he has nothing to do, and said "I wish I had a car so I could get out easier."

O: Client seen in his home and taken on city bus for community reintegration following discharge from inpatient facility. Client demonstrated home management skills and ability to care for animals by simulation. Client was able to identify which bus to catch to go to grocery store, but needed reassurance that his choice was correct. At the grocery store, client chose lunchmeat and fruit for lunches this week, but needed SBA for payment.

This therapist identified the following areas of progress/problems/potential:
Problems:
- Client is anxious about whether his bus choice is really correct.
- Client is still unable to manage money independently.
Progress:
- Client is able to simulate care of home and animals.
- Client is able to choose the correct bus to get to the grocery store.
- Client is willing to choose healthier foods at the store this visit.
Potential:
- In this therapist's professional judgment, the progress shown to date is also a good indicator of rehab potential for this client. She writes her assessment of the data as follows:

A: Client's ability to demonstrate home and animal care activities as taught earlier shows good progress toward being able to live independently in the community. Client also demonstrates progress in community mobility by being able to identify which bus to take to the grocery store this visit, and in ability to care for self by choosing healthier foods than his former choices of chips and donuts. Anxiety level in selecting the correct bus and need for assistance in managing money continue to limit client's functional independence.

New Information

The assessment section is **not** the place to introduce new data. Do not put anything in your "A" that has not been discussed in the "S" or "O". If you find yourself wanting to make a statement in the "A" that is not supported by the data in your "S" or "O", ask yourself what you might have observed to support the assessment statement. Then decide whether you need to add it to your "S" or "O".

Justifying Continued Treatment

One very useful way of justifying continued OT treatment for your client is to end the "A" with the statement "Client would benefit from. . ." and complete the sentence with a justification of continued treatment that requires the skill of an occupational therapist, based on your observations and assessment. Not every therapist ends the "A" in this fashion, but for purposes of learning we will end the "A" in this way. This helps to make certain that justification for continued treatment is present in the note, and is a good method of setting up the plan. After you are more proficient in writing notes and are certain that your note justifies continued treatment, you may choose to cover this material in the plan instead. Below are some examples:

Resident would benefit from environmental cues to orient him to environment.

JW would benefit from continued instruction in problem solving and anger management techniques needed for successful personal and social relationships.

Client would benefit from further instruction in IADL tasks along with visual perceptual and problem-solving activities.

Jim would benefit from compensatory techniques to differentiate letter shapes needed to progress in reading skills.

Veteran would benefit from activities that encourage trunk rotation to facilitate transfers and dressing skills.

Client would benefit from continued mental health education including recognition of his delusions, need for medication, how it can help him, and why it is essential to his recovery.

Client would benefit from reacher, sock aid, and long-handled shoe horn to aid in LE dressing.

Resident would benefit from skilled instruction in sequencing of tasks to increase safety while performing ADL tasks.

Client would benefit from instruction in energy conservation techniques to perform meal preparation and clean-up.

Child would benefit from continued use of modalities which ↓ sensory defensiveness.

Ending the Assessment

Now we can finish the assessment section of the note we began earlier:

S: Client stated that he gets bored during the day when he has nothing to do, and said "I wish I had a car so I could get out easier."

O: Client seen in his home and taken on city bus for community re-integration following discharge from inpatient facility. Client demonstrated ability to care for home and animals by simulation. Client was able to identify which bus to catch to go to grocery store, but needed reassurance that his choice was correct. At the grocery store, client chose lunchmeat and fruit for lunches this week, but needed SBA for payment.

A: Client's ability to demonstrate home and animal care activities as taught earlier shows good progress toward being able to live independently in the community. Client also demonstrates progress in community mobility by being able to identify which bus to take to the grocery store this visit, and in ability to care for self by choosing healthier foods than his former choices of chips and donuts. Anxiety level in selecting the correct bus and need for assistance in managing money continue to limit client's functional independence. Client would benefit from continued instruction in going to new places in the community and instruction in money management to increase his ability to shop without caregiver support.

The following are examples of what the completed assessment section of your note might look like:

A: *Inability to don prosthesis Ⓘ currently limits Ⓘ in ambulation needed for functional toileting. Client would benefit from additional skilled instruction in use of pulley-like fasteners on prosthesis to allow one-handed closure installed this date.*

A: *Martha is beginning to regain some of the independent living skills she had prior to her recent psychotic episode. Fear, isolation, and decreased activity tolerance slow her progress and are the focus of current treatment. Martha would benefit from continued skilled instruction in self-care skills as well as increased socialization and increased physical activity.*

A: *Mary's use of her left hand as a functional assist 60% of the time continues to limit her independence in self-care and play tasks. She would benefit from more bilateral activities to ↑ use of left hand during play.*

A: *Client's spontaneous actions in groups, willingness to share verbally, and improved dress and hygiene seem to indicate an improved mood this week. Progress also noted in unprompted attendance, which is up this week, from 2/8 to 6/8 groups attended. Goals #1 (assertion) and #2 (communication) are met as of this date. Goal #3 (leisure skills) is continued through discharge, pending formulation of a plan for use of leisure time.*

Justifying Continuation of Services

When you justify the need for continuation of occupational therapy services, it is necessary to document the reason the service must be provided by an OT or OTA rather than by another professional or by nonprofessional personnel.

Occupational therapists provide the following services:
- Evaluate clients, identify problems, establish goals, and develop treatment plans.
- Assess or reassess the effectiveness of adaptive equipment/techniques.

Occupational therapists and occupational therapy assistants provide the following services:
- Modify functional tasks/activities, modify homes or other environmental contexts.
- Modify activities through the use of adaptive equipment/assistive devices.
- Provide and instruct in the use of adaptive equipment; instruct in adaptive techniques.
- Fabricate splints and adaptive devices.
- Provide individualized instruction to the client/family/caregiver.
- Determine that the procedure/equipment used is safe and effective.
- Intervene to prevent safety hazards and unsafe behaviors.
- Teach compensatory skills.
- Improve performance areas through remediation approaches.
- Instruct in energy conservation and work simplification.
- Instruct in joint protection.

Skilled occupational therapy is **not** evident when the OT or OTA provides the following services:
- Continues treatment after goals are reached or no further significant progress is expected.
- Carries out a maintenance program.
- Provides routine strengthening or exercise programs if there is no potential for functional improvement.
- Carries out daily programs after the adapted procedures are in place and no further progress is expected.

- Presents information such as handouts on energy conservation without having the client or caregiver perform the activity.
- Provides service to a client who has poor rehabilitation potential.
- Duplicates services with another discipline.

Wording is critical to documenting the necessity for continuing skilled occupational therapy. The occupational therapist **provides skilled instruction** to clients rather than **assisting** them. For example, an OT may provide instruction in methods of energy conservation and work simplification instead of helping the client to perform a strenuous task. Occupational therapists **design** home programs and occupational therapists or occupational therapy assistants may provide **instruction** in home programs, which will then be carried out by aides and family members.

Why should a third party payer reimburse you to watch a client carry out the home exercise program that he performs daily on his own? However, if you are **evaluating** his ability to do all the components of it correctly, or **modifying** it to compensate for recent progress, then your professional skill is clearly required. Analyze your clinical reasoning and then document the principles and strategies used during a treatment session in justifying the continuation of skilled occupational therapy.

WORKSHEET 7-1

Justifying Continued Treatment

Which of the following require the skill of an occupational therapist?

_____ Evaluation of a client.

_____ The practice of coordination and self-care skills on a daily basis.

_____ Establishing measurable, behavioral, objective, and individualized goals.

_____ Developing intervention plans designed to meet established goals.

_____ Analyzing and modifying functional tasks/activities through the provision of adaptive equipment or techniques.

_____ Determining that the modified task is safe and effective.

_____ Carrying out a maintenance program.

_____ Teaching the client to use the breathing techniques he has learned while performing his ADL activities.

_____ Providing individualized instruction to the client, family, or caregiver.

_____ Modifying the intervention plan based on a reevaluation.

_____ Reevaluating a client's status.

_____ Providing specialized instruction to eliminate limitations in a functional activity.

_____ Developing a home program and instructing caregivers.

_____ Making changes in the environment.

_____ Teaching compensatory skills.

_____ Gait training.

_____ Intervening with clients to eliminate safety hazards.

_____ Presenting information handouts (such as energy conservation) without having the client perform the activity.

_____ Routine exercise and strengthening programs.

_____ Adding instruction in lower body dressing techniques to a current ADL program.

_____ Teaching adaptive techniques such as one-handed shoe tying.

_____ Preparing a problem list that identifies present status and potential capabilities.

Remember that the justification for continued treatment must support the frequency and duration of the plan. If the last sentence of your "A" reads, *Client would benefit from information on energy conservation techniques,* do not expect the payer to approve more than one more treatment session.

If this is your last session, complete the sentence with your discharge plan. For example:

> *Client would benefit from continued PROM provided by restorative aide.*

> *Client has been instructed in home exercise program and has demonstrated ability to perform correctly.*

> *Client would benefit from adaptations to the home.*

Mrs. W.'s Stroke

Molly W. is a 62-year-old woman who had a stroke 3 weeks ago. She lives with her husband of 30 years in a one story home. Her husband works full time as an account manager at a local bank. She has good return in her involved lower extremity, and is getting some return in her UE as well. She intends to return home to live with her husband, and will be alone during the day while he is at work. You met Mrs. W. in Chapter 5 when you chose a subjective statement for her treatment session.

> ***S***: *Client says she has difficulty moving* ®️ *UE, although she does not know why it will not move. She reports "It really doesn't hurt. It's just tight."*

> ***O***: *Client seen in rehab gym for UE activities to ↑ AROM in* ®️ *shoulder, activity tolerance, UE strength, and dynamic standing balance, in order to ↑ independence in ADL activities.*

> ***ADL***: *Client seen in room for instruction in safety techniques and adaptive equipment use in toileting. Client needs bilateral grab bars in bathroom to sit → stand safely. Client attempted to stand while pulling on walker and one grab bar. Client was instructed on safety issues and the use of bilateral grab bars.*

> ***Performance skills***: *Client sit → stand CGA for balance. Client worked on activity tolerance, dynamic standing balance and ↓ AROM in right shoulder by moving canned goods from counter to cupboard for 5 minutes before needing a 2-minute sitting rest. After resting, participated in activities to ↑ dynamic standing balance by pouring liquid from a pitcher while standing CGA for balance. After a 1-minute rest, client continued activities to dynamic standing balance and safety in ADL activities by pushing wheeled walker while picking up objects from the floor with a reacher.*

> ***Client factors***: *AROM in right shoulder abduction <90°. PROM right shoulder abduction WNL.*

How would you assess this information? Go back and look at the suggestions given earlier in the chapter, then organize your thoughts by identifying the problems, progress, and rehab potential you see in this client's treatment session today.

What **problems** can you identify? Safety risks? Performance areas not WFL that occupational therapy might impact? Do you see evidence of **progress**? Is there any indication of the client's **rehab potential**? What would this client benefit from? Identify problems, progress, and rehab potential below before reading further to learn how the treating therapist assessed this note.

Mini-Worksheet 7-2: Organizing Your Thoughts

Problems

Progress

Potential

In preparing an assessment of the data in this note, this therapist assesses two main **problem** areas: the safety of transferring to and from the toilet, and the client factors that were not WFL. This therapist was particularly concerned about the safety issues and addressed those first. She also noted the rehabilitation **potential** that would be helpful to a reviewer in deciding whether the client's progress is sufficient to warrant the expense of treatment.

> **A**: *Safety concerns (impulsivity, ↓ dynamic standing balance) noted when client attempts to transfer sit → stand during toileting. Client verbalized an understanding of safety instructions and has potential to progress to independence.*

Next she addressed the clinical reasoning behind devoting time to addressing client factors, in the light of her rehab potential.

> **A**: *Safety concerns (impulsivity, ↓ dynamic standing balance) noted when client attempts to transfer sit → stand during toileting. Client verbalized an understanding of safety instructions and has potential to progress to independence.* **Client's ↓ AROM in right shoulder, ↓ activity tolerance, and ↓ dynamic standing balance all interfere with ability to complete ADL tasks safely and independently.**

She completes the assessment by justifying continued treatment.

> **A**: *Safety concerns (impulsivity, ↓ dynamic standing balance) noted when client attempts to transfer sit → stand during toileting. Client verbalized an understanding of safety instructions and has potential to progress to independence. Client's ↓ AROM in right shoulder, ↓ activity tolerance, and ↓ dynamic standing balance all interfere with ability to complete ADL tasks safely and independently.* **Client would benefit from ℞ UE AROM and strengthening exercises along with continued skilled instruction in safety issues and energy conservation techniques.**

In this case, the therapist decided that the client factors could be addressed in two different ways, both by working on ↑ AROM, strength, and activity tolerance, and by teaching some energy conservation strategies.

We know that payment for ongoing treatment of range and strength is often denied. In Chapter 8 you will see how this therapist plans to provide the things this client would benefit from in a cost-effective manner.

Helpful Hint
Assessment is the "heart" of your note. If you could write only six lines, the assessment section of your note would contain the six lines you would choose. This is the section that demonstrates your clinical reasoning as an occupational therapist.

Assessing Factors Not Within Functional Limits

Some notes will show **progress** and/or rehab **potential**, and some will not, but almost all notes will show **problem** areas, because the problems are what keep a client in active treatment. The most common problem area that you will be assessing is the impact of an underlying factor such as a performance skill or client factor that is not within functional limits (WFL). When therapists are first learning to write SOAP notes, they may find it difficult to distinguish observations from assessments. There is a formula you can use to write about a problem area that is not WFL, insuring that you are writing an assessment rather than an observation. This formula calls for making the limiting factor the subject of the sentence, and then telling how that factor impacts a client's functional ability in a particular area of occupation.

Underlying Factor	Impact	Ability to Engage in Occupation

For example:
- **Deficits in UE strength and activity tolerance** limit client's ability to complete basic self-care tasks.
- **Lack of forearm supination and active elbow flexion against gravity** interfere with child's ability to perform age-appropriate developmental play activities.
- **Pain in Ⓛ shoulder** limits client's ability to carry out child-care and household management tasks.
- **Deficits in attention span** make IADLs difficult and possibly unsafe.
- **Inability to manage anger** results in difficulty finding work and establishing successful intimate relationships.
- **Decreased strength and AROM** interfere with client's ability to transfer and to propel w/c Ⓘ.

Notice that in each of the examples given above, the performance skill or client factor that is not WFL is the subject of the sentence, and then is followed by the negative impact it has on a specific area of occupation. This is not the only way to write an assessment of problem areas, but the formula given is a good one to use when you are first learning.

WORKSHEET 7-3

Assessing Factors Not WFL

You will be rewriting some assessment statements to make them more effective using the following formula:

Underlying Factor	Impact	Ability to Engage in Occupation

For example, this statement is an observation:

> *Client's activity tolerance for lower body dressing was <2 minutes secondary to SOB from asthma.*

It tells you what the therapist observed while providing intervention. To make it into an assessment statement, you would need to change the emphasis by turning your sentence around and by adding the impact the client's SOB has on her independence in dressing. Using the formula above you might write:

> *Client's SOB and activity tolerance of <2 minutes is insufficient for dressing her lower body.*

Rewrite the following statements using the formula given above.

Client demonstrated difficulty with laundry and cooking tasks due to memory and sequencing deficits.

Decreased level of arousal noted during morning dressing activities, requiring redirection to task.

Client unable to follow hip precautions during morning dressing due to memory deficits.

Client problem-solved poorly while performing lower body dressing, as evidenced by multiple attempts to button pants and don socks.

From Borcherding S. *Documentation Manual for Writing SOAP Notes in Occupational Therapy, Second Edition.*
© 2005 SLACK Incorporated

WORKSHEET 7-4

Ellie's Development

Ellie was born prematurely at 24 weeks gestation. She is currently 5 months old. She was referred to OT while in NICU for stimulation of a normal developmental sequence, and continues to receive occupational therapy because she is considered a high-risk infant.

> **S**: *Parent reports that infant is gaining ~1 oz per day and will probably be able to discontinue O_2 in "a couple of days".*

> **O**: *Infant seen in living room of home to assess visual skills and to ↑ mobility skills (head righting, sitting, rolling supine → sidelying and push-up in prone). Infant oriented to black and white illuminated design by turning head. Infant demonstrated visual tracking in horizontal plane 20° past midline. Infant unable to sit, roll, right head, or push up in prone (I), but with facilitation and force of direction technique infant could perform activities after about 20 seconds and hold position. Infant became fatigued and "fussy" after 20 minutes of treatment with four 1-minute rest breaks.*

How would you assess this information? What **problems** can you identify? Are there any factors not WFL that occupational therapy might impact? What influence do the limiting factors above have on Ellie's ability to engage in occupation that is appropriate for her age?

Do you see evidence of **progress**? Is there any indication of Ellie's rehab **potential**? What would she benefit from? After you identify problems, progress, and rehab potential, write an assessment to add to the "S" and "O" given above.

The therapist who is working with Ellie was concerned about the following:
- Inability to perform age appropriate mobility skills (I)
- Became fatigued after 20 minutes
- Lack of head righting response
- Needs O_2

She was encouraged by the following:
- Need for O_2 is decreasing and she is gaining weight
- Ability to hold a position if facilitated
- Ability to orient to a black and white image and to track horizontally

    A:

WORKSHEET 7-5

Ms. D.'s Social Skills

Ms. D. is a 35-year-old woman who has a diagnosis of bipolar disorder, although in a prior admission she was diagnosed with schizophrenia. One of her goals is to talk to the mental health center staff about her problems rather than acting out her feelings. Today she was seen in social skills group with five other clients who also need help with relationship issues.

S: Client reports that she understands the purpose of social skills group. She expressed a desire to attend all the groups, saying that they are "fun."

O: Client seen on the unit for a group session on friendship. Client appeared unkempt, with hair not combed and shirt rumpled. Client engaged in conversation with the other clients and the facilitator. Client interrupted others on 5 occasions. Client spontaneously verbalized her experiences with past friendships and her ideas of useful ways to make new friendships, but had to be redirected to the topic twice during discussion.

What **problems** do you see in the above "S" and "O"?

What areas of occupation do these problems impact?

What evidence of **progress** and/or **potential** do you see?

Write your assessment below:

A:

From Borcherding S. *Documentation Manual for Writing SOAP Notes in Occupational Therapy, Second Edition.*
© 2005 SLACK Incorporated

Chapter 8
WRITING THE "P"—PLAN

The last section of a SOAP note is the **plan**. In this section, you set forth the specific interventions that will be used to achieve the goals. The plan should relate to the information presented in the "O" and the "A," and to your assessment of what the patient would benefit from. It will inform the reader of your priorities regarding intervention strategies. In this book, you will learn to end the "P" with a goal. This is not the only correct way to write a plan, but it is the one we will be using. The choice of what kind of goal to use depends on the facility. In a practice setting where notes are written monthly, your goal would be what you hope to accomplish in the next month. In an acute care setting, it would be your goal for tomorrow.

In an initial evaluation report, this section will contain both the long- and short-term goals, as well as the frequency and estimated duration of treatment. In a contact note or a progress note, you will address any part of the plan that has not been covered in the last sentence of your assessment, "Client would benefit from…." You will address how often you will see the client, how long intervention will continue, and your priorities for what you will work on next. You will end this section with either your long-term goal or your short-term goal, whichever is appropriate to your treatment setting. Goals are always written in measurable, objective, behavioral terms, and include a function and a time line, just as you learned in Chapter 4.

Client will _____ _____ _____
             (action verb)   (skill)   (under what conditions)

_____ _____.
(for what function or occupational gain—if not already indicated)   (by when)

Examples of a "P" might include:

Resident to be seen for 2 more weeks for ½ hr. b.i.d. sessions for skilled instruction in meal/ snack preparation and clean-up. By anticipated discharge on 8/13/05, resident will be able to prepare a TV dinner in the microwave ⓘ at w/c level.

Child will continue to be seen 2x wk. for ½ hour sessions in order to ↑ fine motor skills for better classroom performance. Child will be able to cut a curved line ⓘ within ¼ inch 3/3 tries by the end of the school year.

Client will continue to be seen in groups 5x wk. for 1 week to work on assertion skills and anger management. Pt will demonstrate ↑ social participation by attending 75% of groups without prompting and will spontaneously participate in discussion >5 times by 9/2/05.

Consumer will continue sheltered workshop program 5 days/wk. in order to ↑ work skills. Consumer will attend to task for 60 minutes with no verbal cues within 1 week in order to ↑ ⓘ as a worker.

Continue 1 hour daily sessions for 1 week. Within 1 week, veteran will demonstrate the ability to put arms in holes of shirt 50% of the time after set up with <3 verbal cues.

> Helpful Hint
> If for some reason you are not able to see your client as scheduled, the "plan" section of your note should allow another therapist to continue treatment uninterrupted.

Planning for the Note on Mrs. W.'s Stroke

Now let us write a plan for the note on Mrs. W. that we assessed in the last chapter. As you recall from Chapter 7, Mrs. W. is a 62-year-old woman who had a stroke 3 weeks ago. She has good return in her involved LE and is getting some return in her UE as well. She intends to return home to live with her husband, and will be alone during the day while he is at work.

S: Client says she has difficulty moving ® UE, although she does not know why it will not move. She reports "It really doesn't hurt. It's just tight."

O: Client seen in rehab gym for UE activities to ↑ AROM in ® shoulder, activity tolerance, UE strength, and dynamic standing balance, in order to ↑ independence in ADL activities.

ADL: Client seen in room for instruction in safety techniques and adaptive equipment use in toileting. Client needs bilateral grab bars in bathroom to sit → stand safely. Client attempted to stand while pulling on walker and one grab bar. Client was instructed on safety issues and the use of bilateral grab bars.

Performance skills: Client sit → stand CGA for balance. Client worked on activity tolerance, dynamic standing balance and ↓ AROM in right shoulder by moving canned goods from counter to cupboard for 5 minutes before needing a 2-minute sitting rest. After resting, participated in activities to ↑ dynamic standing balance by pouring liquid from a pitcher while standing CGA for balance. After a 1-minute rest, client continued activities to ↑ dynamic standing balance and safety in ADL activities by pushing wheeled walker while picking up objects from the floor with a reacher.

Client factors: AROM in right shoulder abduction <90°. PROM right shoulder abduction WNL.

A: Safety concerns (impulsivity, ↓ dynamic standing balance) noted when client attempts to transfer sit → stand during toileting. Client verbalized an understanding of safety instructions and has potential to progress to independence. Client's ↓ AROM in right shoulder, ↓ activity tolerance, and ↓ dynamic standing balance all interfere with ability to complete ADL tasks safely and independently. Client would benefit from UE AROM and strengthening exercises along with continued skilled instruction in safety issues and energy conservation techniques.

Write your plan for this client on the next page. Begin with a statement about how often (b.i.d., daily, 2x wk., etc.) and for how long (for 3 days, for 2 weeks, for 1 month, etc.) she will be treated. Look at the items above that she would benefit from, and set your priorities. End with a correctly written goal.

```
┌─────────────────────────────────────────────────────────────────┐
│              Mini-Worksheet 8-1: Plan                             │
│  P:                                                               │
│                                                                   │
│                                                                   │
│                                                                   │
│                                                                   │
│                                                                   │
└─────────────────────────────────────────────────────────────────┘
```

Completing the Plan for Mrs. W.

In assessing the data, the therapist has set up the plan for this note. She has already justified the main things she intended to do and indicated the client's rehabilitation potential. Now she needs to be specific about how often the client will be treated and for what length of time. She first specifies the frequency and duration of treatment.

> **P**: *Continue to treat client 5x wk. for 1 week...*

She could have specified the length of the treatment sessions, i.e., for 1 hr. sessions, but this therapist chose not to do that in this particular note. Next she specifies how she plans to use the treatment time:

> **P**: *Continue to treat client 5x wk. for 1 week **for skilled instruction in safe transfers and toileting**.*

Since she anticipates discharge in 1 week, she has to prioritize her time. She chooses to work on balance and energy conservation as a part of functional mobility and ADL activities. Since she has already written that the client would benefit from additional AROM and strengthening exercises, she now needs to specify how she plans to address this need.

> **P**: *Continue to treat client 5x wk. for 1 week for skilled instruction in safe transfers and toileting. **Home program for AROM and strengthening exercises for Ⓡ shoulder will be taught**.*

This therapist has also indicated clinical reasoning in planning for discharge in advance of the discharge date. In later notes, she will indicate the client's progress in learning the home program. Simply handing the client a set of printed exercises is not considered a billable service. The client's progress in learning the home program will also confirm the therapist's assessment that the client's rehabilitation potential was on target. She will end this plan with a measurable, action-oriented, time-limited goal. Notice that she has specified the conditions under which this action will be carried out.

> **P**: *Continue to treat client 5x wk. for 1 week to work on safe transfers and toileting. Home program for AROM and strengthening exercises for Ⓡ shoulder will be taught. **Client will demonstrate ability to transfer to toilet safely with CGA and use of walker and grab bars by the end of 5 tx. sessions**.*

This note is now complete.

Numbering the Short-Term Goals

Some therapists provide each short-term goal with a number. For example:

STG #1: Resident will prepare a TV dinner in the microwave Ⓘ at w/c level by discharge on 8/13/05.

STG #2: Resident will clear his place setting and wash dishes Ⓘ by 8/13/05.

In notes to follow the therapist can refer to those numbered goals, providing a clear indication of the progress achieved. For example:

A: STG #1: Met. STG #2: Resident requires min Ⓐ to maneuver w/c around table in kitchen and place w/c in appropriate location to reach sink, wash dishes, and put away in cabinets while seated in w/c.

P: Resident will continue skilled instruction in meal preparation until anticipated discharge in 1 week. At the time of discharge, resident will be Ⓘ in all meal prep and clean-up while seated in w/c.

WORKSHEET 8-2

Completing the Plan for Baby Ellie

Now it is your turn. In the last chapter, you wrote an assessment for a treatment note on Ellie's development. Now you will have the opportunity to complete that note by adding a plan. In the last sentence of your "A", you have established a general outline of what you want to do.

In your "P", state how often you plan to see Ellie, how long each session will last, how long you plan to continue your intervention before reevaluating or discontinuing treatment, and how you plan to use your time. End your plan with a functional, measurable, action-oriented, time-limited goal.

As you recall from Chapter 7, Ellie is a 5-month-old infant who was born prematurely at 24 weeks gestation. She was seen in the NICU, and continues to receive OT in her home because she is considered a high-risk infant.

S: Parent reports that infant is gaining ~1 oz per day and will probably be able to discontinue O_2 in "a couple of days".

O: Infant seen in living room of home to assess visual skills and to ↑ mobility skills (head righting, sitting, rolling supine → sidelying and push-up in prone). Infant oriented to black and white illuminated design by turning head. Infant demonstrated visual tracking in horizontal plane 20° past midline. Child unable to sit, roll, right head, or push up in prone Ⓘ, but with facilitation and force of direction technique infant could perform activities after about 20 seconds and hold position. Infant became fatigued and "fussy" after 20 minutes of treatment with four 1-minute rest breaks.

A: Need for facilitation and force of direction techniques limit infant's ability to perform early mobility skills. Limited mobility combined with her tolerance for less than 20 minutes of activity limits her ability to explore her environment and reach developmental milestones at a typical age. Ability to perform mobility skills with facilitation techniques and decreasing need for O_2 both show progress. Orientation to black and white design and ability to track in horizontal plane show good potential for increased environmental interaction and developmental gains. Infant would benefit from continued occupational therapy services to stimulate developmental skills and from parent education in a home program.

P:

WORKSHEET 8-3

Completing the Plan for Ms. D.

As you recall from Chapter 7, Ms. D. is a 35-year-old woman who has a diagnosis of bipolar disorder, although in a prior admission she was diagnosed with schizophrenia. One of her goals is to talk to the mental health center staff about her problems rather than acting out her feelings. Today she was seen in social skills group with five other clients who also need help with relationship issues.

You have noted in the last sentence of your assessment some of the areas of intervention that you think might benefit Ms. D. Now you will fill in the specifics of your plan.

> **S**: *Client reports that she understands the purpose of social skills group. She expressed a desire to attend all the groups, saying that they are "fun."*

> **O**: *Client seen on the unit for a group session on friendship. Client appeared unkempt, with hair not combed and shirt rumpled. Client engaged in conversation with the other clients and the facilitator. Client interrupted others on 5 occasions. Client spontaneously verbalized her experiences with past friendships and her ideas of useful ways to make new friendships, but had to be redirected to the topic twice during discussion.*

> **A**: *Client's unkempt appearance, interrupting behaviors, and need for redirection to topic of conversation interfere with her ability to engage in social participation with peers. Her expressed interest in groups, her willingness to engage in conversation and share her ideas show good potential to develop relationships and to express herself verbally in place of acting out. Client would benefit from attending groups stressing conversational skills and attention to social cues, and from assistance with ADL activities stressing hygiene and appearance.*

> **P**:

Chapter 9
INTERVENTION PLANNING

Now that you know the basics of writing a SOAP note, we will back up a little and give some attention to the intervention planning on which your notes are based. In *Guidelines for Documentation of Occupational Therapy* (AOTA, 2003), the intervention plan is considered one of the three process areas of common reports, the other two being the evaluation and the outcomes. The intervention plan is described as including the long-term functional goals; short-term goals; the intervention or treatment procedures; the type, amount, frequency, and duration of treatment; and recommendations for other services or specialized treatments (AOTA, 2003).

Your critical thinking as an occupational therapist is more evident in the development of the intervention plan than anywhere else in your work. The intervention plan is a creative work in progress. It is a dynamic, creative, joint venture between you and your client (along with the family or significant other when appropriate), and is oriented toward the client's ultimate success in fulfilling his life roles. The intervention plan must be realistic; that is, it must have a good chance of success in a reasonable period of time. It must show evidence of the need for your professional skill. The intervention plan must be discussed with the client, and together you and the client must create this plan for achieving the client's rehabilitation goals and for enabling his ability to engage in meaningful occupation.

The Process

From the moment the referral is received, intervention planning begins in the mind of the therapist. A name, age, and reason for referral will stimulate a good occupational therapist to begin reviewing in his mind the areas of occupation he is likely to assess, the areas of deficits he might expect to find, and the possible interventions he might want to use. Each individual is different of course, and there will be many variations, as well as some surprises as he begins the assessment. The mental preparation for *"Angus Campbell, age 68, Ⓛ CVA, evaluate and treat"* takes a therapist on a mental journey along one road of thought, whereas *"Lindsey Johnson, age 4, ADHD"* takes the therapist mentally down a different pathway. From day one, a good therapist also begins discharge planning based on the client's occupational profile, prior level of functioning, and probable discharge placement.

As soon as the order is received, the therapist documents the referral in the health record and reviews the available information about the client in preparation for his first visit. The information may be obtained from the health record or a call to the physician or a conversation with the teacher who made the referral. It is helpful to know the answers to questions that have already been asked by other health professionals, rather than asking them again.

The next step is a visit to the client. In an outpatient setting, much information is gleaned from simply watching the client enter into the treatment area. Does the client guard for pain? Is a supportive family member accompanying the client? What is the quality of movement and posture? Are there obvious cognitive or perceptual problems?

If the client is oriented and verbal, an interview is first on the agenda. If the client is not able to provide information, the family or other caregiver may be able to provide the information needed. What is the occupational profile of this client? What areas of this client's life present the most problems? What was the client able to do prior to this injury or hospitalization? What roles are important to this client? What does this client desire from treatment? What results does the family hope to see? What supports are available to facilitate the desired results?

From this interview, the therapist begins selecting evaluation tools. First, it is important to evaluate areas of occupation and then underlying factors (performance skills and patterns, context, activity demands, and client factors). In this way, no time will be lost evaluating underlying factors that do not impact ability to engage in meaningful occupation (Youngstrom, 2002b).

The initial evaluation leads to formulation of a problem list. The therapist and client agree on the priorities for treatment for this client at this time. This leads directly to setting goals and choosing treatment interventions. It is also important to know who is paying for your services (Lloyd, 2004). Workers' compensation programs are state-supported programs funded by employers to provide for services for a person injured on the job. Therefore, the covered services revolve around treatment focused on the person's ability to return to work. Medicare, on the other hand, is a federally funded insurance program mainly for persons over the age of 65 and provides primarily for the treatment of acute illnesses that result in deficits in self-care. Its recipients are usually retired.

In the public school system where therapy services are mandated by federal laws such as IDEA and where some of the therapy services are funded by Medicaid, occupational therapy treatment must be educationally relevant treatment that focuses only on the child's functioning in the classroom. Private insurance organizations such as Blue Cross may provide for coverage of services for a wider variety of goals than other payers or may cover occupational therapy only for narrower and more specific treatments for certain diagnoses. All payers, however, are interested in the amount of time that will be needed for intervention and in the cost-effectiveness of the intervention provided.

Documentation of the initial evaluation is provided in whatever format the facility uses. Most practice settings use forms for initial evaluation reports. An example of such a form is found in Chapter 10. The initial evaluation may be handwritten or computerized. It may be a narrative note or a SOAP note. Although initial evaluations are quite lengthy and time-consuming when written in the SOAP format, the information gathered in an initial evaluation fits nicely into the SOAP format.

S: The interview data.
O: The evaluation data from both standardized evaluation tools and your clinical observations.
A: Your professional assessment of the data you reported in "O"; your determination of the rehab potential and the problem list.

From the **S, O,** and **A,** the goals and objectives are established, leading to:

P: Frequency and duration of treatment, along with the intervention strategies for meeting the goals and objectives.

Estimating Rehabilitation Potential

Rehab potential is always stated as good or excellent for the goals you want to accomplish. If it is not good or excellent for your client, select a smaller, more incremental goal. There is not much point in setting and working toward goals that you do not have a good chance of accomplishing. Estimating rehab potential as poor, fair, or guarded is a red flag to reviewers and they may be reluctant to set aside health care dollars for someone who is unlikely to benefit. Rehab potential does not mean independence. It means potential to reach the goals you have set or potential for the client to make significant change.

Selecting Intervention Strategies

Since selecting strategies and treatment media is a daily task for an occupational therapist, it can seem to an inexperienced therapist almost like reinventing the wheel to select these differently for each individual client. One of the striking differences between occupational therapy and other disciplines is the way in which strategies and media are selected to meet the client's goals. In occupational therapy, the task must be meaningful to the individual client, and selected for its meaningfulness (Youngstrom, 2002b). Occupational therapy is a process of creative problem solving with each client in each area of occupation. What is meaningful to one client may not be to another.

Even the most basic task such as dressing may not seem meaningful to some clients. A person with tetraplegia who has a personal attendant, for example, may never need to dress himself, and may consider it an enormous waste of time to be required to learn to do so. However, he may be very motivated to learn to hold a cue stick in order to reengage in social participation with his friends. Some clients will never need to balance a checkbook while others may not be able to return to living independently without this skill. The difference between competent and exceptional occupational therapy may well lie in the ability to find meaningful activities and design these into intervention strategies.

The occupational therapist asks questions like these:

- What do you want to be able to do?
- What keeps you from being able to do that?
- What are the possible options for making that happen?

The options for intervention strategies may include teaching new skills or patterns, working to increase client factors (range, strength, and endurance), or modifying the environment (context). Occupational therapists consider doing things in many different ways. The creativity of the individual therapist blossoms in intervention planning. How many ways are there to get light into a room if the client can no longer manage a light switch? How many activities that require wrist extension could be adapted to reach the objective of increasing AROM at the wrist needed to return to work on the assembly line? Would any of these qualify as meaningful to this client?

The treatment media used by occupational therapy is also different from that used by other disciplines. Occupational therapists often use common household objects to accomplish functional tasks. For example, the client's own clothing is a common treatment media. The clothes may be used for dressing to teach the client to don clothing or may be used for folding in order to be doing a meaningful activity while increasing standing tolerance, or for hanging in a closet to increase AROM at the shoulder. The approach would depend upon what the client will need to do in the setting to which she will be discharged. An experienced occupational therapist can find many different uses for common household objects. The same net ball that is used to wash dishes may be used for squeezing to develop grip strength or for throwing to develop AROM in the upper extremities.

Developing Intervention Strategies

Intervention strategies do not stand alone. Strategies must be based on problems and long-term goals, and they must be purposeful to the client to be useful. However, for the purpose of learning to generate possible strategies, we will suspend that requirement and think of as many ways as possible to meet a treatment objective. Consider the following example:

STG	Interventions
Client will be able to complete basic ADL tasks while standing for 5-minute increments and taking rest breaks as needed by discharge date 9/10/05.	1. *Set up task to make coffee while standing at counter in the ADL kitchen.* 2. *Instruct client to stand at the bathroom sink to wash hands after toileting.* 3. *Instruct client to stand in a standing table to play a game.* 4. *Instruct client to stand to arrange clothing while dressing in the AM.* 5. *Instruct client to stand to look out window to watch birds eat the food she has put out.*

WORKSHEET 9-1

Choosing Intervention Strategies

Using the short-term goal below, think of as many intervention strategies as possible that would help the client meet his goal.

STG	Intervention Strategies
Client will be able to manage his financial affairs ① *in order to live alone after discharge.*	

Contents of the Intervention Plan

The format of the intervention plan will vary from one facility to another. In this manual, you will see more than one format for creating an intervention plan. Since the intervention plan is technically a part of the initial evaluation report rather than a document that stands on its own, how much of the demographic and referral data is recorded on the intervention plan itself and how much is recorded elsewhere in the evaluation report varies from one practice setting to another. Somewhere in the health record it is necessary to record targeted outcomes based on the evaluation report, and the intervention strategies and approaches that will be used to achieve these outcomes. The *Guidelines for Documentation of Occupational Therapy* (AOTA, 2003) state that the intervention plan should include:

- Basic demographics or client information.
- Goals and objectives.
- Intervention approaches to be used.
- The mechanism for delivering services, including frequency and duration of treatment.
- The discharge plan.
- Methods for measuring the success of the outcomes.
- Names/positions of the persons responsible for carrying out the plan.
- Date the plan was developed, reviewed, or modified.

Frequency and Duration of Treatment

Under a managed care reimbursement system, a set number of visits will be approved. A therapist must learn to set priorities that will use the approved time to the client's best advantage. When negotiating for the number of visits to be allowed, it is useful to make a sound case for what you want, backed up by reasons and probable results, and based on the rehab potential. In a practice setting where therapy is based on an already established formula of treatment minutes, you will also need to prioritize your treatment goals.

It can sometimes seem impossible to a new therapist to estimate how much time will be needed to accomplish goals. With a little experience you will find that you really can do it. Please remember that the intervention plan is made to be changed. If your original estimate does not turn out to be accurate, you change it as you find out how quickly your client progresses.

Next we will look at an example of an evaluation and intervention plan containing the consumer's long- and short-term goals and possible intervention strategies that might be used. For purposes of demonstration, the plan used as an example covers only one problem, although this would be unusual in a real treatment setting.

Intervention Plan

Client Name: *Marge B.*   **Age**: *71*   **Sex**: *F*   **Health Record #** *04136*
Primary Diagnosis: Ⓛ *CVA*   **Secondary Diagnosis**: *Diabetes*
Referring Physician: *F. Dittrich, M.D.*   **Date of Treatment Plan**: *12/21/05*
Frequency and Duration of Treatment: *2x day for 3 weeks (30 treatment sessions)*
Primary Occupational Therapist: *Charlet Quay, OTR/L*

Occupational Profile: *Ms. B. is a widow who lives with her daughter and grandson in a one-story house in a small town. Ms. B. was* Ⓘ *in all ADL and IADL tasks before her CVA. She has never worked outside her home. She raised 7 children in the town where she now resides and takes pride in her ability to do homemaking tasks such as cooking, sewing, and decorating. She drives in her own small town, but is not comfortable driving long distances. She intends to return to the home she shares with her daughter and grandson, and expects to return to her PLOF.*

Problem: *Client requires mod* Ⓐ *in self-care due to inability to spontaneously use* Ⓡ *UE 2° * Ⓛ *CVA.*

Long-Term Goal: *Client will be able to complete self-care and IADL activities* Ⓘ*within 3 weeks.*

STG (Objective)	Interventions
STG #1 *Client will demonstrate spontaneous use of* Ⓡ *UE as a functional assist in self-care within 1½ weeks.*	1. *Normalize tone through the use of NDT approaches.* 2. *Instruct in sensory stimulation to affected side to ↓ neglect.* 3. *Weight bear on* Ⓡ *UE while engaged in functional activities that require weight shifts: sorting laundry, playing a board game, turning pages of a magazine.* 4. *Facilitate grasp and release for use of prehension; facilitate reach patterns through handling, joint approximation, guided resistance, and muscle stretch.* 5. *Provide activities that require* Ⓡ *UE as an assist (stabilizing tablet while writing, stabilizing toothpaste while removing lid) or* Ⓑ *UE use (wringing out washcloth, applying body lotion).*

STG #2 *Client will dress self with min Ⓐ within 2½ weeks using Ⓡ UE as a functional assist.*	*1. Instruct in adaptive dressing techniques.* *2. Instruct in use of Ⓡ UE to stabilize shirt while buttoning, assist in pulling up pants, holding on to bra while hooking in front.* *3. Instruct in adaptive equipment as needed: long shoe horn, elastic shoelaces, reacher, or dressing stick.* *4. Facilitate trunk control and balance in weight shifts forward and backward, side to side, and in rotational patterns in preparation for and throughout dressing activity as needed.*
STG #3 *Client will be safe in light meal preparation and clean-up with SBA in 3 weeks.*	*1. In collaboration with client and family, adapt kitchen for safe accessibility and mobility.* *2. Plan meal with attention to money management, organization, and sequencing of component tasks.* *3. Instruct in functional mobility in kitchen to transport items while preparing lunch using gait patterns learned in PT. Use wheeled cart as needed for efficient and safe transport of items.* *4. Instruct in correct and safe body mechanics in reaching items in refrigerator, on stove top, in oven or microwave, and in performing sink, countertop, and cooking activities.* *5. Instruct in energy conservation during meal preparation and cleanup.* *6. Select and instruct in use of appropriate adaptive equipment for one-handedness as needed to peel and chop vegetables, open cans and jars.*

In the next worksheet, you will have an opportunity to combine several of the skills you have learned so far. You will have the demographic data, the beginning of an occupational profile, and the subjective and objective data from an evaluation. It will be up to you to:

- Assess the data, as you learned in Chapter 7.
- Write problem and goal statements, as you learned in Chapters 3 and 4.
- Determine priorities for treatment and decide on frequency and duration of treatment, as you learned in Chapter 8.
- Write an intervention plan, as you learned in this chapter.

WORKSHEET 9-2

The Case of Ginny H.

Name: *Ginny H.*　　**Age**: *87*　　**Sex**: *F*　　**Physician**: *B. Garrett, M.D.*
Diagnoses: Ⓛ *subdural hematoma on 4/22/05, hx. of hypertension, hearing loss*
Onset: *4/22/05*　　**Date of Referral**: *5/2/05*　　**Date of Evaluation**: *5/3/05*
Referral Source: *Nursing on 5/2/05*

Background data and beginning occupational profile: *Prior to her stroke Ginny had been living for the last 10 years with her unmarried daughter, Sue, who is 60 years old and works full-time. They live in a two-story house with a bathroom on the second floor. Ginny was in acute care and has just been discharged to a rehabilitation program. She expresses a desire to return to her daughter's home. Her daughter has concerns about being able to care for her mother at home. Ginny has Medicare insurance only.*

S: *Client expressed frustration when having difficulty brushing teeth. Client c/o back pain 2/10 when grooming. Client's daughter said that client was* Ⓘ *in self-care prior to her stroke but has not cooked or done housework for years; further stated client has a hearing loss but no hearing aids.*

O: *Client seen in room for initial assessment.*

Dressing/Grooming: *Client stood with CGA for 5 min while brushing teeth after setup and 2 verbal cues. Client* Ⓘ *in donning/doffing socks with extra time. Client continued to attempt to don* Ⓡ *sock using the same techniques for several minutes before being successful. Client did not attempt an alternative technique. Client mod* Ⓐ *in donning/doffing gown and robe due to difficulty pulling the robe around her back and threading the* Ⓡ *UE into the sleeve. Client required four 30-second rest breaks during dressing activity due to fatigue.*

Transfers/Ambulation: *Client sit → stand with SBA and mod* Ⓐ *for transfer ↔ bedside commode due to ↓ standing balance when managing clothing. Client walked 3 ft. w/c → sink with CGA using walker.*

UE ROM & Strength: *All UE AROM was WNL except for* Ⓑ *shoulder abduction and flexion which were WFL.* Ⓑ *UE strength 5/5 overall except 3/5 in shoulder flexion and abduction.*

Lateral Pinch (lb.): Ⓡ *7.5;* Ⓛ *9. Tripod pinch (lb.)* Ⓡ *4;* Ⓛ *7.*

Grip (lb.): Ⓡ *29;* Ⓛ *37.*

Sensation: *Light touch and sharp/dull tests indicated intact sensation* Ⓑ*. Client correctly identified 1/4 objects in the* Ⓡ *stereognosis test.*

Coordination: *9 hole peg test: Placing pegs* Ⓡ *52;* Ⓛ *37. Removal* Ⓡ *26;* Ⓛ *14*

Write an assessment for this data, as you learned to do in Chapter 7. Turn your problems into correctly worded problem statements. Identify the rehab potential you see for Ms. H. On the intervention plan, you will include some of these items as "strengths".

A:

Now complete the treatment plan.

From Borcherding S. *Documentation Manual for Writing SOAP Notes in Occupational Therapy, Second Edition.*
© 2005 SLACK Incorporated

Frequency and Duration of Treatment:

Strengths:

Functional Problem Statement #1:

Long-Term Goal #1

STGs (Objectives)	Interventions

Functional Problem Statement #2:

Long-Term Goal #2

STGs	Interventions

Using Groups to Provide Interventions

In some practice settings, clients are seen primarily in groups rather than individually. This strategy has the advantage of using peer feedback and support as a part of the treatment process. It also provides challenges for the therapist in finding ways to structure the group to meet the needs of all the clients attending. Next we will consider a client who is being seen in a psychiatric unit where intervention strategies generally take place in groups. After you read about this client, you will be choosing some intervention strategies to use for her in each of the groups she attends.

Sarah's Suicide Attempt

Sarah J. is a 40-year-old, unemployed, psychiatrically disabled woman who recently separated from her husband. She has two children, a daughter age 22 and a son age 18. Sarah was admitted through the emergency department post ingestion of an overdose of psychiatric medications. She was lavaged, and admitted briefly to a medical unit, where she was stabilized in 8 hours and transferred to psychiatry with a diagnosis of depression.

Sarah was sexually abused from the ages of 10 to 13 by an uncle who lived in the home where she was one of five children. Her estranged husband abuses alcohol and is emotionally abusive to Sarah when he has been drinking. Sarah married him when she was 18 years old and pregnant with her first child. They have been married for 21 years.

Sarah reports that she has trouble with expression of anger. She doesn't always know she is getting angry, and then "explodes" in ways that are destructive to herself, others, and property. She also says that she is having a lot of trouble making decisions, and that her husband has traditionally made decisions for her. She says that she "just can't think" and has difficulty paying attention to anything for more than a few minutes. For example, she is unable to complete a magazine article she is reading. Her appearance is disheveled, her hair is uncombed, and she is wearing no makeup or jewelry. She picks at her clothing while she talks to you, looking at the floor and making little eye contact.

The problem areas identified by the treatment team include anger, decision making, and poor self-esteem with suicidal ideas. Sarah's anticipated length of stay is 4 days. The psychiatric unit provides an array of individual and group treatment sessions.

In addition to the medication group and the individual sessions done by the psychiatrist, there is group therapy provided by the social worker, and an evening wrap-up group provided by nursing. Occupational therapy provides three groups per day.

- Goals group ½ hour each morning
- Stress management group 1 hour daily
- IADL group 1 hour daily

The IADL group covers such topics as money management, parenting, assertion skills, and other IADL skills as desired, depending on the needs of the group. You plan this group around the issues that are common to the clients currently attending. For example, if several clients have difficulty expressing anger in useful ways, you could use the IADL group time to address anger management.

In a psychiatric unit, the treatment plan is usually multidisciplinary. We will discuss multidisciplinary treatment plans in Chapter 11. Because we are working with a 4-day length of stay, and a multidisciplinary treatment plan, we will not write objectives for each of Sarah's goals. Sarah will be seen in occupational therapy groups every day while she is in the hospital. In the next worksheet, you will decide how to use the group time to Sarah's best advantage in meeting her established goals. Keep in mind that your interventions will include not only the activities you plan to use, but also the ways you plan to use yourself as a therapeutic agent with Sarah—the ways you might plan to interact with her and the behaviors you might want to model.

WORSHEET 9-3

Planning Interventions for Sarah

Problem #1: Exacerbation of depression including low self-esteem and a recent suicide attempt, leading to safety concerns in an independent living environment.

LTG #1: By anticipated discharge in 4 days, Sarah will demonstrate an increase in self-esteem by a neat appearance, making eye contact during conversation at least once daily, and verbally identifying a positive resource or coping strategy she has used successfully in the past.

> Interventions:
> Goals Group
>
> Stress Management Group
>
> IADL Group

Problem #2: Stress related to recent role changes result in Sarah's inability to focus her thoughts sufficiently to make decisions for her daily life.

LTG #2: Sarah will have a plan in place for making decisions regarding her two most important current life decisions by discharge in 4 days.

> Interventions:
> Goals Group
>
> Stress Management Group
>
> IADL Group

Problem #3: Sarah does not recognize anger building and does not have useful ways of expressing it, resulting in expressions of anger that damage self, relationships, and property.

LTG #3: By anticipated discharge in 4 days, Sarah will identify feelings, behaviors, and bodily sensations that are associated with varying stages of anger.

> Interventions:
> Goals Group
>
> Stress Management Group
>
> IADL Group

The Critical Care Pathway

In response to the changing health care payment systems, many facilities have developed a form of a standardized intervention plan called a critical care pathway. Certain kinds of illnesses, surgeries, and disabilities follow a predictable course of recovery. The body responds in a similar way to the condition, even though each person's experience will be unique. Critical care pathways are part of overall quality improvement efforts in health care facilities. In striving for quality care in the most cost-effective manner, the focus of health care is on the outcomes of that care and on the major components that are involved in the delivery of the care.

The goals of critical care pathways and the other monitoring involved in quality improvement programs are to provide some predictability in outcomes, to establish a system of integrating care provided by a myriad of disciplines, and to allow for comparative analysis of treatment and treatment settings. The format of the pathways allows for monitoring a client's progress on a comparative basis.

In addition to standardizing intervention strategies and establishing check points along a time line, the use of a standard intervention plan also is more efficient by avoiding unnecessary time spent in rewriting basically the same plan for routine treatment approaches. The standardized plan does allow for adaptations to accommodate individual client differences such as multiple diagnoses.

Critical care pathways are usually established to be multidisciplinary but may be specific to occupational therapy. In a setting like a skilled nursing facility that primarily has clients with Medicare insurance coverage, the interventions and client education provided by each discipline is usually designed to be completed in an allotted number of days that are established by the Diagnostic Related Grouping (DRG) system. An orthopedic unit in an acute care hospital may establish the number of days of treatment based on a retrospective analysis of the hospital's health records of orthopedic hospitalizations.

Critical Care Pathways in Rehabilitation

Some diagnoses such as CVA are too complex to use a standardized approach to treatment. Other diagnoses such as a total hip replacement are very compatible with the critical care pathway system. A critical care pathway for a client with a total hip replacement might resemble the example in Table 9-1.

Table 9-1
Critical Care Pathway—Total Hip Replacement

Day 1 (admission to rehab, post surgery)
- Initial evaluation
- Film on total hip precautions
- Review precautions and have client demonstrate to insure understanding

Day 2
- Skilled instruction in functional mobility while following hip precautions
- Assess, provide, and instruct in necessary adaptive equipment
- Begin UE strengthening
- Begin ADL training (dressing, grooming, hygiene)

Day 3
- Continue UE strengthening
- Continue ADL training
- Skilled instruction in tub and shower transfers
- Introduce home program and have client demonstrate to insure understanding

Day 4
- Skilled instruction in car transfers and stair climbing
- Home evaluation for safety
- Reassess client's understanding of home program

Day 5
- Discharge

Common Errors in Writing Intervention Plans

Problem Identification

- Problems identified in the assessment are not addressed in the plan.
- Problems are not stated in terms of behavioral manifestations, area of occupation, and underlying factors.
- The number of visits or units requested does not match the severity of the problems.

Goals

- Goals are not functional or do not focus on the reason for admission to occupational therapy.
- Intervention plan does not focus on specific rehabilitation goals that will increase a client's ability to engage in meaningful occupation in the probable discharge environment.
- Goals focus on the client participating in or cooperating with treatment (unless the client is in the habit of refusing treatment).
- Goals cannot be measured or do not have a target date for completion.

Treatment Interventions

- Interventions do not focus on increasing functional behaviors in order to return the client to the least restrictive environment.
- Interventions do not take into account the age, sex, and interests of the client or are not meaningful to the client.
- Acquired skills are not transferred into more functional contexts in a client's life.

Client Involvement

- The client is not involved in the treatment planning process. The client's signature on the intervention plan indicating that client has read it is not enough to indicate significant client involvement.
- Intervention plan does not reflect the client's strengths, desires, and preferences.

Canned Plans

- "Canned" intervention plans reflect the same goals, objectives, and interventions for each client based on the services available rather than on client need. Even critical pathways need to be individualized to fit the client.

Chapter 10

Documenting Different Stages of Treatment

As we discussed in Chapter 1, different stages of the intervention process require occupational therapists to write different kinds of notes. Very early in the process, an **intake note** may be written acknowledging the referral and stating a plan to evaluate. Next, a screening or **evaluation report** is written, containing the client's occupational profile and current concerns and priorities as well as the assessment results. From this comes the **intervention plan**, which outlines the specific areas of occupation that will be addressed and the outcomes expected. Facilities vary in the type and frequency of **contact** or **progress notes** required. Some settings require a contact note (also called a **treatment note** or **visit note**) for each visit. Others may require a **progress note** every week or every 30 days, and more frequently for new referrals or for a change in status. The requirements for type and frequency of notes are usually a function of the service setting, the accrediting agency, and the payment source. Sometimes a **reassessment note** is required at regular intervals. If a client is transferred from one setting to another within the same service delivery system, a **transition plan** may be written. Most facilities require a **discharge or discontinuation report** at the end of treatment to summarize the occupational therapy services provided and the changes in a client's ability to engage in meaningful occupation as a result of occupational therapy intervention.

In actual practice, you will find that contact, progress, and reassessment notes may have some overlap. For example, in outpatient settings the contact notes often include the client's progress. Contact notes in settings where clients may change quickly, such as acute care, may also read much like progress notes. In some ways, progress notes reassess the client's status and may sound much like reassessment notes. Notes may also be named differently or combined in some service delivery systems. There are guidelines for each kind of note, however, and in this chapter we will examine the requirements for documentation at each stage of client care.

In *Guidelines for Documentation of Occupational Therapy* (AOTA, 2003), criteria for notes in three process areas are described: evaluation, intervention, and outcome. Evaluation and screening reports, along with reassessment reports are considered **evaluations**. The intervention plan, contact notes (also called treatment notes or visit notes), progress reports, and transition plans are a part of the **intervention** process. Discharge or discontinuation notes record professional activity in the area of **outcomes**.

There are some essential elements that must be present in all documentation. These include:
- Client's name and case number
- Date and kind of contact
- Identification of type of documentation, agency, and department
- Signature and credentials of person providing service
- Countersignature of student notes (and on OTA notes if required by law or facility)

In addition, medical terminology used must be appropriate to the setting, errors must be corrected with one line and the therapist's initials, and the therapist must adhere to professional standards regarding technology, timelines for documentation, disposal and storage of records, and compliance with HIPAA standards for confidentiality. In the following exercises, we will compare some notes to the AOTA criteria that have been set for them, and see how well the notes stand up under scrutiny.

Initial Evaluation Reports

After a referral for occupational therapy is received on a client, you begin gathering information about the client's occupational profile. You will need to know the client's occupational history, as well as what factors impact engagement in occupation. This is the beginning of the occupational profile, which will tell you what that client needs and wants from occupational therapy. First, you collect data from the client, the family, the chart, and any other pertinent sources. Then you select and administer any standardized tests or survey instruments that will help you determine more exactly what underlying factors support or hinder participation in occupations. From your initial evaluation reports, you will identify and prioritize the areas of occupation and underlying factors that need your attention and develop an intervention plan.

Under the current Prospective Payment System (PPS) used by Medicare in long-term care settings, the time spent in initial evaluation is becoming shorter in order to allow for treatment to begin sooner, and impacting the amount of data that is initially collected. Our challenge as we move further into the 21st century is to be as complete as we can in evaluating a client in the amount of time we have to complete the evaluation.

Most facilities provide a form for an initial evaluation report, and evaluation results are recorded on the form, along with comments and observations. Some facilities use the same form for reevaluation and discharge reports so that the evaluation material does not have to be rewritten. Figure 10-1 shows the evaluation/reevaluation/discharge report form from Capitol Region Medical Center in Jefferson City, Missouri so that you can see what might be included on a good facility form. Because this is an acute care facility, there is an emphasis on some areas of occupation (ADL) over others (such as play or social participation). If you are writing an initial evaluation as a SOAP note, this is the way you would categorize your information.

S: The interview material

O: The tests results and clinical observations

A: Your professional assessment of the data presented in the S and the O

P: Frequency and duration of planned interventions and the long- and short-term goals

There are many correct ways to format the information, and different facilities may choose to organize the information any way they like as long as it is all present. Several different formats are used in this manual to make it clear that there is no one "correct" organizational strategy.

CAPITAL REGION MEDICAL CENTER
OCCUPATIONAL THERAPY
☐ **INITIAL EVALUATION** ☐ **DISCHARGE SUMMARY**

DIAGNOSIS _____ ONSET: _____

MED. HX: _____

_____ CODE STATUS: _____

RELEVANT SURG. PROC.: _____

REFERRAL DATE: _____ DATE: _____

REFERRING PHYSICIAN: _____ MEDICARE #: _____

ACTIVITIES OF DAILY LIVING REHAB POTENTIAL: _____

DRESSING Put on & remove the following	INDEP	SBA	MIN. ASSIST	MOD. ASSIST	MAX. ASSIST	ADAPT. EQUIP.	COMMENTS/ADAPTIVE EQUIPMENT ISSUED
front opening shirt							
pull on shirt							
underwear							
bra							
pants/slacks							
socks/hose							
shoes							
manage fasteners							
braces/splints/prosthesis							
GROOMING/HYGIENE							
sponge bath							
tub/shower bath							
shave							
comb hair							
brushing teeth							
opens jars/bottles							
make-up							
EATING							
drink from cup/glass							
feeds self							
cuts meat							

UPPER EXTREMITY ROM & STRENGTH

ROM ACTIVE LEFT	PASSIVE LEFT	ACTIVE RIGHT	PASSIVE RIGHT			STRENGTH L	R
				SHOULDER:	Elevation		
					Flexion		
					Abduction		
					Horizontal Abduction		
					Horizontal Adduction		
					Internal Rotation		
					External Rotation		
				ELBOW:	Flexion		
					Extension		
					Supination		
					Pronation		
				WRIST:	Flexion		
				Shoulder Subluxation	L	R	
				UE Edema	L	R	
				Pain	L	R	

PERTINENT FINDINGS

Wears glasses_____ Dentures_____ Hearing_____

MUSCLE TONE/UPPER EXTREMITIES

Hypotonic_____ Normal_____ Hypertonic_____
Comments_____

UPPER EXTREMITY SENSATION

SENSATION	Intact	Impaired	Absent
Light touch			
Sharp/Dull			
Temperature			
Proprioception			
Stereognosis			

COORDINATION/UPPER EXTREMITIES

Tremors_____ Apraxia_____ Ataxic_____

	Impaired	WNL
Gross Motor		
Fine Motor		
9 Hole Peg Test	L	R
Grip Strength	L	R
Lateral Pinch	L	R
Tripod Pinch	L	R
Hand Dominance	L	R

SURVIVAL SKILLS	Indep.	Min. Assist	Mod. Assist	Max. Assist
Phone Book Usage				
Money Mngmt.				
Situational Problem Solving				
Homemaking				

ORIENTED TO:

Person_____ Place_____
Time: Month_____ Day_____ Year_____
Situation_____

COMMUNICATION/COGNITION

	YES	NO
Verbal		
Understandable		
Appropriate		
Perseveration		
Follows Simple Commands		
Reads		
Writes		

PERCEPTION

A. R/L Neglect_____

	Impaired	WNL
B. Body Schema		
C. Discrimination		
Shape		
Size		
Color		
D. Visual Perception		

Overall Endurance WFL_____
Fair_____
Poor_____

2,605,003 (9/99) INIT. EVAL/DISCHG. SUM. (FRONT)

Figure 10-1a. Occupational therapy initial evaluation and discharge summary form (page 1). Courtesy of Capital Region Medical Center, Jefferson City, MO.

HOME SITUATION:_____

LIVING ARRANGEMENTS: (PT ADDRESS) _____

HOME TYPE:_____

PRIOR FUNCTIONAL INDEP.: _____

_____

_____

LEISURE INTERESTS: _____

ADAPTIVE EQUIP.:_____

COMMENTS:_____

_____

_____

_____

PATIENT / FAMILY GOALS:_____

❑ INITIAL ASSESSMENT (PROBLEMS / STRENGTHS)   ❑ DISCHARGE STATUS OF SHORT / LONG TERM GOALS

_____

_____

_____

_____

_____

PLAN:_____

SHORT-TERM GOALS - ESTIMATED TIME TO ACHIEVE: _____

_____

_____

_____

_____

_____

❑ LONG-TERM GOALS - ESTIMATED TIME TO ACHIEVE: ❑ RECOMMENDATIONS:

_____

_____

_____

_____

_____

_____

❑ Yes   ❑ No   **Patient has participated in evaluation process and agrees with treatment plan as stated above.**

        Therapist _____   Date_____

I have reviewed and agree with the treatment plan as stated above.

        Physician Signature _____   Date_____

2,605,003 (9/99) OT INITIAL EVALUATION/DISCHARGE SUMMARY (BACK)

Figure 10-1b. Occupational therapy initial evaluation and discharge summary form (page 2). Courtesy of Capital Region Medical Center, Jefferson City, MO.

The *Guidelines for Documentation of Occupational Therapy* (AOTA, 2003) list the following criteria for the content of an evaluation:

1.   Documents the referral source and data gathered through the evaluation process. Includes:
   a.   Description of the client's occupational profile.
   b.   Analysis of occupational performance and identification of factors that hinder and support performance in areas of occupation.
   c.   Delineation of specific areas of occupation that will be targeted for intervention and outcomes expected.
2.   An abbreviated evaluation process (e.g., screening) documents only limited areas of occupation applicable to the client and the situation.
3.   Suggested content with examples:
   a.   <u>Client information</u>—name/agency, date of birth, gender, applicable medical/educational/developmental diagnoses, precautions, and contraindications.
   b.   <u>Referral information</u>—date and source of referral, services requested, reason for referral, funding source, and anticipated length of service.
   c.   <u>Occupational profile</u>—client's reason for seeking occupational therapy services, current areas of occupation that are successful and areas that are problematic, contexts that support or hinder occupations, medical/educational/work history, occupational history (e.g., patterns of living, interests, values), client's priorities, and targeted outcomes.
   d.   <u>Assessments used and results</u>—types of assessments used and results (e.g., interviews, record reviews, observations, and standardized or nonstandardized assessments), description of the client factors, contextual aspects of features of the activities that facilitate or inhibit performance, and confidence in test results.
   e.   <u>Summary and analysis</u>—interpretation and summary of data as it is related to occupational profile and referring concern.
   f.   <u>Recommendation</u>—judgment regarding appropriateness of occupational therapy or other services.

Reprinted with permission from *Guidelines for Documentation of Occupational Therapy* (AOTA, 2003)

Read the following initial evaluation report and intervention plan. Use the checklist in Worksheet 10-1 to evaluate the report against the criteria described in the *Guidelines for Documentation of Occupational Therapy* (AOTA, 2003). In each square on the right side of the checklist, make a note of how the evaluation meets the criteria.

Occupational Therapy Initial Evaluation Report

Name: Agnes H.   **Age**: 68   **Sex**: F   **Physician**: T. Grantham, M.D.
Date of Onset: 2/1/05   **Date of Admission**: 2/2/05
Referral Data: Client referred by Dr. Grantham for evaluation and treatment.

Occupational Profile: Client was admitted after a fall resulting in confusion and left-sided weakness. Prior to admission she was living alone in a one-story home and was ① in all activities of daily living. Client is a retired librarian and states she values her independence and fully intends to return to her own home. Hobbies include mostly sedentary activities such as sewing, reading, and playing cards with friends. Daughter works for United Wickets, lives two blocks away and is willing to visit daily and assist with transportation, but cannot provide supervision.
1° Dx: Ⓡ CVA r/o OBS   **2° Dx**: Diabetes
Date of Evaluation: 2/3/05   **Time**: 10:00 am

S: Client stated, "I'm doing this so I can go home."

O: Client seen at bedside and in shower room for mini mental status exam, evaluation of personal ADL tasks (toileting, dressing ↔ undressing and showering), functional mobility, and underlying factors (manual muscle test, AROM).

Bathing: Upper body: min Ⓐ to sequence task; Lower body: min Ⓐ except max Ⓐ to reach perineal area and feet.

Dressing: Seated in chair with arms, min Ⓐ to maintain dynamic balance when bending, mod Ⓐ to initiate donning bra, and max Ⓐ to reach feet. Verbal cues needed for sequencing and environmental orientation.

Toileting: Verbal cues to flush, min Ⓐ to obtain tissue and manage clothing.

Transfers: CGA with verbal cues for safety/proper arm placement sit to stand; min Ⓐ from low surfaces.

Bed Mobility: Rolls & supine ↔ sit SBA for safety.

Standing Balance: Static: CGA.

Activity Tolerance: Fair (3) (1-5 scale) <10 min tolerance to any activity with physical/mental challenges.

Motor Planning/Perception: WFL.

Cognition: Score of 17/30 on MME. Sequencing problems during dressing tasks noted. Client could not attach bra in back and required verbal cues to attach in front.

UE AROM: WFLs for all Ⓑ UE movements except: abd, int/ext. rotation of Ⓛ shoulder.

UE Strength: Grip: Ⓡ 42 lbs. Ⓛ 21 lbs. Pinch: Ⓡ palmar 14#; Ⓡ lateral 15#; Ⓛ palmar 6#; Ⓛ lateral 8#.

Manual Muscle Test: All movements 4/5 except Ⓛelbow ext. 3/5, thumb opposition and abduction 3+

Sensation: Ⓛ UE: Light touch, pain, temperature intact; Stereognosis 3/5; Ⓡ UE all intact

A: Client's poor problem-solving skills (trying to doff pants prior to doffing shoes/socks and inability to initiate an alternative way to don bra) and the need for verbal cues to initiate some ADL tasks limit her ability to manage her basic and instrumental ADL activities Ⓘ. Decreased AROM and strength in the Ⓛ UE along with slow response to cognitive tasks, decreased ability to sequence tasks, and decreased short-term memory are safety concerns in an independent living situation. Client would benefit from environmental cues to orient her to environment, facilitation of problem solving, and sequencing activities, and activities to increase strength in the Ⓛ UE. Rehab potential is good for modified Ⓘ in ADL activities.

P: Client will be seen for 45 minute sessions 5x wk. for 2 wks. for sequencing during ADL tasks, problem-solving strategies, activities to increase activity tolerance & strength in Ⓛ UE. Put calendar in client's room to increase orientation to month, day, and season. Evaluate ability to handle emergency situations. Client will be able to dress with SBA and <3 verbal cues after set-up within 2 weeks.

Intervention Plan

Problem #1: Client needs min to max physical assist and verbal cues to dress self due to ↓ AROM, activity tolerance, and ability to sequence the task.

LTG: Client will be able to dress with SBA and <3 verbal cues after set-up within 2 weeks.

STGs	Interventions
Client will don bra Ⓘ using adapted technique within 3 days.	1. Teach adaptive techniques. 2. Post picture of how to don bra correctly using adapted technique. 3. Reinforce correct responses. 4. Teach strengthening program for UE.
Client will don shoes and socks Ⓘ using adapted technique and a long shoehorn within 5 days.	1. Provide long shoehorn and instruct client in correct use. 2. Instruct in adapted techniques for donning shoes and socks. 3. Post picture of adapted technique and long shoehorn being used to don shoes. 4. Instruct in using affected side as a functional assist in dressing. 5. Expand exercise program to include AROM.
Client will sequence dressing tasks correctly 3/3 tries within 1½ weeks.	1. Verbalize steps before beginning to dress. 2. Verbalize steps while dressing. 3. Post list of steps for client to follow. 4. Take rest breaks as needed for activity tolerance.

Problem #2: Client's lack of orientation to environment and inability to problem solve cause safety concerns with ADL and home management.

LTG: When asked, client will correctly use calendar, schedule, clock, and emergency information posted on wall within 2 weeks.

STGs	Interventions
Client will correctly identify time, date, and situation when asked within 1 week.	1. Post calendar, schedule, and emergency information near clock in client's room. 2. Instruct family, nursing staff, and other therapy staff to ask client date, time, and situation several times daily and to reinforce correct responses.
Client will be able to follow a daily schedule with <2 verbal cues within 1½ weeks.	1. Post daily schedule on wall near clock. 2. Cue client to look at schedule to determine what she should be doing at any given time.
Client will correctly problem solve responses to emergency situations with 90% accuracy within 2 weeks.	1. Provide situations for client to problem solve, progressing from easy to more complex. 2. Provide telephone directory or other props as needed for problem solving.

WORKSHEET 10-1

Initial Evaluation Report

How well does the evaluation report for Agnes H. meet the criteria established by AOTA?

Background Data

Criteria	Compliance
Are all of the following present: name, date of birth, gender? What are the applicable diagnoses?	
Who referred the client to OT, on what date, what services requested?	
What is the funding source?	
What length of stay is anticipated?	
Why is the client seeking occupational therapy services?	
Are there any secondary problems, preexisting conditions, contraindications or precautions that will impact therapy?	

Occupational History and Profile

Is there an occupational history/profile? Is it adequate?	
Which areas of occupation are currently successful and which are problematic?	
What factors hinder her performance in areas of occupation? What factors support her performance in areas of occupation?	
What are the client's priorities?	
What areas of occupation will be targeted for intervention? Do these match the client's priorities?	
What are the targeted outcomes?	

Results of the Assessment

What types of assessments were used?	
What were the results of the assessments?	
What client factors, contextual aspects, and activity demands are identified as needing attention?	
What factors (strengths, supports) facilitate her occupational performance?	
How confident is this OT that her evaluation results are valid?	
Is OT appropriate for this client?	

WORKSHEET 10-2

Intervention Plan

The *Guidelines for Documentation of Occupational Therapy* (AOTA, 2003) list the following criteria for the content of an intervention plan:

1. Documents the goals, intervention approaches, and types of interventions to be used to achieve the client's identified targeted outcomes based on results of evaluation or re-evaluation processes. Includes recommendations or referrals to other professionals and agencies.
2. Suggested content with examples:
    a. <u>Client information</u>—name/agency, date of birth, gender, precautions, and contraindications.
    b. <u>Intervention goals</u>—measurable goals and short-term objectives directly related to the client's ability to engage in desired occupations.
    c. <u>Intervention approaches and types of interventions to be used</u>—intervention approaches that include: create/promote, establish/restore, maintain, modify, and prevent: types of interventions that include: consultation process, education process, therapeutic use of activities to enhance occupation, and therapeutic use of self.
    d. <u>Service delivery mechanisms</u>—service provider, service location, and frequency and duration of services.
    e. <u>Plan for discharge</u>—discontinuation criteria, location of discharge, and follow-up care.
    f. <u>Outcome measures</u>—outcomes that include improved occupational performance, client satisfaction, role competence, improved health and wellness, prevention of further difficulties, and improved quality of life.
    g. <u>Professionals responsible and date of plan</u>—names and positions of persons overseeing intervention plan, date plan was developed, and date when plan was modified or reviewed.

Reprinted with permission from *Guidelines for Documentation of Occupational Therapy* (AOTA, 2003)

How well does the intervention plan for Agnes H. meet the AOTA criteria?

Criteria	Compliance
Is client information present on the evaluation or intervention plan (name, age, gender, precautions, contraindications)?	
Are the types of interventions to be used identified?	
Are the intervention goals and objectives measurable?	
Are the goals and objectives directly related to the client's ability to engage in the desired occupations?	

What is the anticipated frequency/duration of services?	
What is the discontinuation criteria?	
What is the anticipated discharge location?	
What is the anticipated plan for follow-up care?	
What is the name and position of the person overseeing the plan of care?	
What date was the plan developed, and what date(s) was it modified or reviewed?	

Contact Notes

Contact, visit, or treatment notes are used to document each visit or each individual occupational therapy session. In some situations, such as home health, contact notes are required in the health record each time a client is seen. In other cases, the occupational therapist keeps attendance records, logs, or informal contact notes, which are used for the purpose of writing a summary of progress.

The *Guidelines for Documentation of Occupational Therapy* (AOTA, 2003) list the following criteria for the content of a contact note:

1. Documents contacts between the client and the occupational therapist or the occupational therapy assistant. Records the types of interventions used and client's response. Includes telephone contacts, interventions, and meetings with others.
2. Suggested content with examples:
    a. <u>Client information</u>—name/agency, date of birth, gender, diagnosis, precautions, and contraindications.
    b. <u>Therapy log</u>—date, type of contact, names/positions of persons involved, summary or significant information communicated during contacts, client attendance and participation in intervention, reason service is missed, types of interventions used, client's response, environmental or task modification, assistive or adaptive devices used or fabricated, statement of any training education or consultation provided, and the persons present.

Reprinted with permission from *Guidelines for Documentation of Occupational Therapy* (AOTA, 2003)

Read the following contact note from an acute care practice setting, and use Worksheet 10-3 to determine how well it meets the guidelines.

Acute Care Unit

Client: John B. **Sex**: M   **Health Record** # *123456*
Date: *4/14/05* **Time**: *8:30 AM*   **Attending Physician**: A. Smith, MD

S: *Mr. B. reports, "I feel fair today. I had a long night."*

O: *Client seen bedside in ICU for instruction in ADL tasks and AROM in Ⓡ UE. Client nodded his head when asked if ready to sit up; required mod Ⓐ supine → sit. Upon sitting O$_2$ saturation dropped to ~85%. Grooming, dressing, and UE AROM activities not completed 2° low O$_2$ levels. Client given min Ⓐ to return to supine. After ~2 minutes O$_2$ levels returned to ~95%. Client washed face p̄ set-up in supine and nodded when asked if that felt good.*

A: *Client able to tolerate a little more activity today than yesterday when he did not have tolerance for supine → sit. Client also appears more motivated to attempt therapy session. Activity tolerance still limited due to O$_2$ saturation levels upon exertion, which limits ability to participate in self-care tasks. Client would benefit from instruction in energy conservation as well as correct positioning to ↓ exertion ↑ activity tolerance for ADL tasks.*

P: *Continue skilled OT daily to ↑ activity tolerance, and Ⓘ in ADL tasks for 5 days or until discharge. Client will complete grooming EOB c̄ rest breaks as needed within 3 treatment sessions.*

Bonnie B., OTR/L

WORKSHEET 10-3

Treatment, Visit, or Contact Notes

How well does the contact note for John B. meet the criteria established by AOTA?

Criteria	Compliance
Is client information (name, date of birth, gender, diagnosis, precautions, and/or contraindications) present?	
What is the date and time of the contact?	
What type of contact is this?	
What are the names and positions of the persons involved in the contact?	
Is there a summary of the intervention or the information communicated during the contact?	
Is the client's participation in the contact (or the reason service was missed) present?	
Is there an indication of the environmental or task modification, assistive or adaptive devices used or fabricated, training, education, or consultation provided, and persons present?	

Progress Notes

Progress notes are written on a regularly scheduled basis (usually weekly or monthly), with the time frame determined by the facility. The facility is guided by the accrediting agencies and primary payers in setting the time frame in which progress notes must be written. The progress note provides a summary of the intervention process and the documents the client's progress toward goals.

The *Guidelines for Documentation of Occupational Therapy* (AOTA, 2003) list the following criteria for the content of a progress note:

1. Summarizes intervention process and documents client's progress toward goals achievement. Includes new data collected; modifications of treatment plan; and statement of need for continuation, discontinuation, or referral.
2. Suggested content with examples:
   a. Client information—name/agency, date of birth, gender, diagnosis, precautions, and contraindications.
   b. Summary of services provided—brief statement of frequency of services and length of time services have been provided; techniques and strategies used; environmental or task modifications provided; adaptive equipment or orthotics provided; medical, educational, or other pertinent client updates; client's response to occupational therapy services; and programs or training provided to the client or caregivers.
   c. Current client performance—client's progress toward the goals and client's performance in areas of occupations.
   d. Plan or recommendations—recommendations and rationale as well as client's input to changes or continuation of plan.

Reprinted with permission from *Guidelines for Documentation of Occupational Therapy* (AOTA, 2003)

Read the progress note that follows and use the checklist in Worksheet 10-4 to evaluate it against the AOTA criteria.

Behavioral Health Center Progress Note

S: In assertion group on Tuesday 10/11/05, client talked about how her life had taken a "downward spiral" since early September, and she had become more passive and less proactive in getting her needs met, although she had not been aware of it at the time.

O: Client attended assertion group 2/2, communication group 1/1, and IADL group 3/5 this week. She was on time to 4/6 groups without reminders, wearing neatly pressed clothing, makeup, and an ornament in her hair. In assertion group on Thursday 10/12 she shared (without prompting) 2 stories about her usual way of dealing with retail situations. In communication group she spontaneously answered one question addressed to the group as a whole, and in IADL group she offered to assist another client with his checkbook.

A: Client's spontaneous actions in groups and willingness to share verbally indicate an improved mood this week. Her unprompted attendance is up this week from 2/8 to 6/8 groups. Her improved dress, hygiene, and makeup also indicate an improvement in mood from last week. Client would benefit from planning a structure for her days to prevent another "downward spiral" after discharge.
Goals #1 (assertion) and #2 (communication) are met as of this date.
Goal #3 (leisure skills) is continued through discharge on 10/15/05 pending formulation of a plan.
Goal #4 (parenting skills) was discontinued on 10/10/05.

P: Client to be seen in groups for 2 more days, with discharge anticipated on Wednesday of next week. IADL group will be used for preparing the structured plan for using her time. Client will prepare a plan including at least one planned leisure activity per day for at least 5 days out of 7 after discharge and will discuss it with her husband and social worker by discharge on 10/15/05.

Sharon A. Young, OTR/L, 10/11/05

WORKSHEET 10-4

Progress Notes

How well does this progress note comply with the criteria set out by AOTA?

Criteria	Compliance
Is client information (name, date of birth, gender, diagnosis, precautions, and/or contraindications) present?	
What is the frequency of services? How long have services been provided?	
What techniques and strategies were used? What programs or training were provided to the client or caregiver?	
Were any environmental or task modifications provided? Any adaptive equipment or orthotic devices?	
What other pertinent client updates are given?	
What is the client's response to occupational therapy services?	
What is the client's progress toward her goals?	
What areas of occupation are being addressed?	
What recommendations are made and why? What is the client's input to changes or continuation of the intervention plan?	

Reevaluation Reports

In some practice settings, clients must be reevaluated monthly or quarterly. In others, reevaluation is done as needed. The reassessment report is rather a cross between a progress note and a discharge summary, which documents the results of the reevaluation process. The tests that were given initially are readministered, and the results are compared with the results of the previous tests to determine the effectiveness of the treatment being provided. The goals and plans are revised at this time and new time lines are projected.

The *Guidelines for Documentation of Occupational Therapy* (AOTA, 2003) list the following criteria for the content of a reassessment note:

1. Documents the results of the reevaluation process. Frequency of reevaluation depends on the needs of the setting and the progress of the client.
2. Suggested content with examples:
   a. Client information—name/agency, date of birth, gender, applicable medical/educational/developmental diagnoses, precautions and contraindications.
   b. Occupational profile—updates on current areas of occupation that are successful and problematic, contexts that support or hinder occupations, summary of any new medical/educational/work information, and updates or changes to client's priorities and targeted outcomes.
   c. Reevaluation results—focus on reevaluation, specific types of assessments used and client's performance and subjective responses.
   d. Summary and analysis—interpretation and summary of data as related to referring concern, and comparison of results with previous evaluation results.
   e. Recommendations—changes to occupational therapy services, revision or continuation of goals and objectives, frequency of occupational therapy services, and recommendation for referral to other professionals or agencies where applicable.

Reprinted with permission from *Guidelines for Documentation of Occupational Therapy* (AOTA, 2003).

Read the reevaluation report that follows and use Worksheet 10-5 to determine how well it meets the AOTA criteria.

Hand Clinic Reevaluation Report

Name: Jane P. **DOB:** 5/12/64   **Sex**: Female
Primary Diagnosis: Osteoarthritis of the CMC joints bilaterally
Secondary Diagnosis: None   **Precautions/Contraindications**: none
Referring Physician: R. Oliver, MD   **Date of Referral**: June 27, 2005
Reason for Referral: Client is 1 month postsurgery (LRTI) to the Ⓛ CMC joint and carpal tunnel release
Date of Initial Evaluation: 7/5/05   **Date of Reevaluation**: 8/31/05
Funding Source: University insurance

Occupational Profile: Jane is a 41-year-old Caucasian female who works as an administrative assistant in the English Department at the University. She lives alone in a small, two-story farmhouse 7 miles outside of town. The house is heated with wood that Jane cuts and stacks in the summer. Jane raises a large vegetable garden every year, in addition to holding both a full-time job at the University and a part-time job in a department store. She began experiencing pain in the CMC joints of both hands approximately 3 years ago. She intends to continue her present living arrangement and both of her jobs.
She was originally admitted to the outpatient hand clinic on July 5, 2005 at 1 month postsurgery for hand rehabilitation following a successful LRTI and a carpal tunnel release. She is being re-evaluated this date (8/31/05) to determine whether further occupational therapy services are needed.

S: *Client initially reported continuous pain at a level of 3/10 and pain on overexertion of the hand at a level of 5/10, resulting in irritability and difficulty performing bilateral work and daily living tasks, as well as some tasks requiring left hand use. On this date, she reports no continuous pain and pain at a level of 1/10 when typing for more than 45 minutes without rest breaks.*

<u>Initial ability to engage in work/ADL/IADL tasks (by client report):</u>

- *Unable to use keyboard with all fingers of (L) hand. Types with one finger on standard keyboard.*
- *Unable to grasp cylindrical objects smaller than 1½ inches (broom handle, toothpaste tube) due to ↓ AROM.*
- *Unable to wear watch or rings on (L) hand due to swelling.*
- *Unable to turn door knob with (L) hand to enter house when right hand is full.*
- *Unable to lift laundry basket and other items requiring (B) UE use. Unable to lift purse or other items needed for IADL tasks c̄ with left hand.*

<u>Current ability to engage in work/ADL/IADL tasks this date (by client report):</u>

- *Able to use new ergonomic keyboard for primary work task using all fingers.*
- *Able to sweep the floors with a regular broom.*
- *Able to fold laundry using (B) hands.*
- *Able to grasp small items needed for ADL and IADL tasks (toothpaste tube, key, lids) but not at PLOF.*
- *Able to turn doorknob if door is unlocked.*
- *Able to hang out clothes on clothesline, including carrying basket and holding garments with left hand.*

  O:

Initial evaluation of client factors 7/05/05	*Reassessment of client factors 8/31/05*
Total active motion of the wrist: 125°	*Total active motion of the wrist: 160°*
Total active motion of the thumb: 110°	*Total active motion of the thumb: 130°*
Grip strength (R) 41#	*Grip strength (R) 40.7#*
Grip strength (L) 15# (31% of (R))	*Grip strength (L) 22.6#*
Pinch not tested	*Pinch not tested*
Some edema	*No edema*

Client has been seen in outpatient hand clinic for three 45-minute visits since admission on 7/05/05. Active and passive range of motion have been performed, taught to client, and home program has been modified as she progressed. Heat has been used, and the client has purchased a home paraffin unit. Electrical stimulation (10%) has been used to elicit specific motion and facilitate strengthening of the flexor pollicus longus. A strengthening program has been added to the HEP, and client is able to demonstrate all HEP exercises correctly. Client has received education on the structure and use of the hand, common features of carpometacarpal (CMC) arthritis, ergonomics of the workstation, energy conservation, use of heat for pain relief, and adapted techniques for ADL activities. Client reports understanding the education, and has been given written material covering the same content.

A: *Increase in grip strength of 7# shows good progress in strength needed to perform functional tasks. Thumb AROM is now WFL, and wrist AROM is increased 35° to 80% of average, allowing client to perform most work and ADL tasks (I) in ways that do not damage the joint. Change to an in ergonomic keyboard and understanding and correct self-administration of HEP indicate good potential to continue improvement without continued occupational therapy services.*

P: *Client to call hand clinic if questions arise, and follow the home program of heat, exercise, and adapted techniques. Results of reevaluation indicate no further need for occupational therapy services unless new problems arise.*

Brad E., OTR/L, CHT

WORKSHEET 10-5

Reevaluation Reports

How well does the reevaluation note on Jane's hand rehabilitation meet the AOTA criteria?

Criteria	Compliance
Is client information (name, date of birth, gender, diagnosis, precautions, and or contraindications) present?	
What is the updated status of current areas of occupation that are successful or problematic?	
What contexts support occupations? What contexts hinder occupations?	
Is there a summary of any new medical/work/educational information?	
What are the updates/changes to the client's priorities and targeted outcomes?	
What was the focus (purpose) of the reevaluation?	
What assessments were used?	
How do the results compare with the previous evaluation results?	
What is the client's response to the reevaluation?	
Is there an interpretation of the summary and comparison of results with previous evaluation results?	
What changes to occupational therapy services, goals, or referrals will be made as a result of the re-evaluation?	

From Borcherding S. *Documentation Manual for Writing SOAP Notes in Occupational Therapy, Second Edition.*
© 2005 SLACK Incorporated

Transition Plans

A transition plan is written whenever a client transfers from one setting to another within a service delivery system. It is designed to provide information to the new service providers so that care is uninterrupted. Transition plans summarize the client's current occupational status, specify what service setting the client is leaving, state what setting she is entering, and tell how and when the transition will occur.

The *Guidelines for Documentation of Occupational Therapy* (AOTA, 2003) list the following criteria for the content of a transition plan.

1. Documents the formal transition plan and is written when client is transitioning from one service setting to another within a service delivery system.
2. Suggested content with examples:
   a. <u>Client information</u>—name/agency, date of birth, gender, diagnosis, precautions, and contraindications.
   b. <u>Client's current status</u>—client's current performance in occupations.
   c. <u>Transition plan</u>—name of current service setting and name of setting to which client will transition, reason for transition, time frame in which transition will occur, and outline of activities to be carried out during the transition plan.
   d. <u>Recommendations</u>—recommendations and rationale for occupational therapy services, modifications or accommodations needed, and assistive technology and environmental modifications needed.

Reprinted with permission from *Guidelines for Documentation of Occupational Therapy* (AOTA, 2003).

Read the transition plan for Julie M. and use the checklist in Worksheet 10-6 to determine how well it meets the AOTA criteria.

Transition Plan

Name: Julie M.   **Date of Birth**: 4/29/02   **Gender**: Female
Date of Plan: April 11, 2005   **Expected Transition Date**: May 2005
Precautions/Contraindications: Seizure disorder
Occupational History: Julie experienced head and orthopedic injuries following a MVA at 9 days of age. Since that time she has had multiple cranial, hip, and leg surgeries. She is currently under the management of a neurologist as well as an orthopedist. The mother carries out a home program daily which is designed to stimulate development.

S: The mother reports that although Julie's seizures, multiple surgeries, and illnesses have slowed her development, the family is hopeful that Julie will progress more rapidly through her developmental milestones now that the surgeries are finished and the seizures are under control.

O: Child received her first occupational therapy screening in the hospital 1 week postinjury. She received formal developmental assessments at 2, 4, 6, 12, and 24 months of age. Parents were given home program following the initial formal assessment. Regular OT treatment sessions were started at 12 months of age and have continued to this date. Child has been seen twice weekly in her home and monthly in the Birth-to-Three clinic. She is now eligible, due to her age, for preschool services.

<u>Current occupational performance</u>: Current problems being treated in occupational therapy include visual regard and visually directed reach, midline orientation, postural symmetry, and motor overflow. Current goals for Julie include functional reach, grasp and release, rolling, and ability to sustain antigravity positions for ADL and developmental play activities.

A: At 3 years of age, Julie is at about a 4-month level of development. Although the mother provides a stimulating environment, Julie would benefit from continuation of regular occupational therapy, physical therapy, and speech therapy services to facilitate her continued progress through the developmental sequence.

P: Julie will receive her first preschool service evaluation next month in May 2005. Parents have been given a home program, which has been updated as child has progressed in treatment. Home program will continue through the transition to preschool services.

WORKSHEET 10-6

Transition Plan

How well does the transition plan for Julie meet the criteria established by AOTA?

Criteria	Compliance
Is client information (name, date of birth, gender, diagnosis, precautions, and/or contraindications) present?	
What is the client's current performance in occupations?	
What is the current setting?	
What is the setting into which the client is transferring?	
What is the reason for the transition?	
What is the time frame in which the transition will occur?	
What activities are to be carried out during the transition plan?	
What recommendations are made for occupational therapy services in the new setting?	
What is the rationale for this recommendation?	
What modifications, accommodations, assistive technology, or environmental modifications are needed?	

Discharge Summaries

A discharge summary (also called a discontinuation report) is used to summarize the changes in the client's ability to engage in occupation and to make recommendations for referral or follow-up care if needed. Discharge notes often follow a format of their own, stating the date and purpose of the referral, giving a summary of the initial findings, the course of treatment, a summary of progress and any recommendations for follow-up care. Discharge summaries may be done as S.O.A.P. or narrative notes, or the facility may have a particular form that is used. Some facilities use the same form for evaluation, reevaluation and discharge, making it quicker to prepare the discontinuation report.

The *Guidelines for Documentation of Occupational Therapy* (AOTA 2003) list the following criteria for the content of a discharge report:

1. Summarize the changes in the client's ability to engage in occupations between the initial evaluation and discontinuation of services and make recommendations as applicable
2. Suggested content with examples:
    a. Client information—name/agency, date of birth, gender, diagnosis, precautions, and contraindications.
    b. Summary of intervention process—date of initial and final service; frequency, number of sessions, summary of interventions used; summary of progress toward goals; and occupational therapy outcomes – initial client status and ending status regard ing engagement in occupations, client's assessment of efficacy of occupational therapy services.
    c. Recommendations—recommendations pertaining to the client's future needs; specific follow-up plans, if applicable; and referrals to other professionals and agencies, if applicable.

Reprinted with permission from *Guidelines for Documentation of Occupational Therapy* (AOTA, 2003).

The discontinuation note we will be evaluating in Worksheet 10-7 is written in a SOAP format, and then offered again written as it might appear on a facility form, so that you can see it done both ways.

Occupational Therapy Discharge Summary

Occupational Therapy Note   **Date**: 2/19/05   **Time**: 3:00 PM

S: Client reports that she is very pleased with the outcome of her occupational therapy treatment, and with her ability to take care of herself at home. She reports no steps to the front entrance of a one story home, and no architectural barriers inside the house. She reports that she owns the following adaptive equipment already: wheeled walker, reacher, dressing stick, sock aid, long shoehorn, tub bench, raised toilet seat, and grab bars around the toilet and in the tub.

O: Client seen bedside and in clinic area 20/20 sessions from SOC on 1/25/05.

ADL status on 1/25/05	ADL status on 2/19/05
Mod Ⓐ in transfers	SBA in transfers
Mod Ⓐ in toileting	Ⓘ in toileting
Mod Ⓐ in feeding	SBA in feeding after set-up
Mod Ⓐ in dressing	Dressing from arm chair requires set up only, but SBA for standing and pulling pants up over hips
Max Ⓡ for safety in bathing	SBA in bathing with min Ⓐ w/c ↔ shower using tub bench.

Client education in adaptive techniques and HEP were discussed with client and client demonstrated ability to perform correctly. Home modifications discussed with client and caregiver.

A: *Client has made good progress in self care activities and shown by differences in admitting and discharge abilities. Since caregiver is available to provide SBA needed for safety in ADL tasks, all treatment goals have been met, and client is ready for discontinuation of occupational therapy services.*

P: *Client to continue home exercise program. Adaptive equipment recommended: walker basket and reacher holder for walker. Client and caregiver to decide how to implement home modifications. Client to continue outpatient physical therapy. No direct occupational therapy services recommended at this time.*

Now let us consider the same discharge note, written on a form provided by the rehabilitation facility:

Rehabilitation Center

Discharge Note

Occupational Therapy Note   **Date**: *2/19/05*   **Time**: *3:00 PM*

Course of Rehabilitation: *Client seen 20/20 sessions from SOC on 1/25/05. Skilled instruction in adaptive techniques for ADLs provided. Client progress was good and she met all tx. goals. Client now requires SBA in all transfers, lower body ADLs, upper body ADLs, grooming/hygiene. She is Ⓘ in toileting. Client also requires SBA in feeding after setup. Dressing from arm chair with wheeled walker, set-up only but SBA for standing and to pull pants up over hips. Bathing is SBA with min Ⓐ w/c ↔ shower using tub bench.*
Client Education: *Recommendations for additional adaptive equipment and modifications to home discussed with client and caregiver. Client and caregiver were instructed in home exercise program of theraband, free weights, wands, and other activities to choose from for Ⓑ UE strengthening. HEP discussed with client and client demonstrated ability to perform exercises correctly.*
Discharge Recommendations/Referrals: *Discharge with home caregiver. Continue home exercise program. Adaptive equipment recommended: walker basket and reacher holder for walker. Client already has wheeled walker, reacher, dressing stick, sock aid, long shoehorn, and functional bathroom equipment and has demonstrated ability to use these correctly and safely. Client will be seen in outpatient PT. No direct OT services are recommended at this time.*
Paul H., OTR/L

WORKSHEET 10-7

Discharge Summary

How well do the discharge summaries above meet the criteria established by AOTA? Does one format meet the criteria better than the other does?

Criteria	Compliance
Is client information (name, date of birth, gender diagnosis, precautions, and/or contraindications) present?	
What was the date of initial service? What was the date of end of service?	
What was the client's progress toward goals?	
What was the client's beginning and ending status regarding ability to engage in occupations?	
What is the client's assessment of occupational therapy services?	
What are the recommendations pertaining to the client's future needs?	

From Borcherding S. *Documentation Manual for Writing SOAP Notes in Occupational Therapy, Second Edition.*
© 2005 SLACK Incorporated

Chapter 11
DOCUMENTATION IN DIFFERENT PRACTICE SETTINGS

In this chapter, we will examine documentation in several different practice situations. Each of these practice settings has some requirements that are specific to the setting or the primary payment source. Documentation for these settings is different in some ways from the examples you have learned so far.

Documentation in Mental Health

If you go from a job in a rehabilitation center to one in a mental health setting, you might think that nothing you have learned about documentation applies. Problems, goals, and interventions are often multidisciplinary and may be written in a different format from what you have learned. The language used in the documentation may seem less specific. Some mental health issues (such as suicide risk or past sexual abuse) may not fit very neatly into the *Framework* (Holmquist, 2004). Also, intervention is often provided in groups or within a therapeutic environment or milieu. Occupational therapy services may be included in a treatment service designated as adjunctive therapy, activity therapy, or expressive therapy, which may include therapeutic recreation specialists, music therapists, art therapists, and dance therapists. Professional roles often overlap and there is often a blurring of professional identities. Reimbursement may not be discipline-specific and therapy services may be included in the room rate for the facility.

One of the exceptions is geriatric psychiatric mental health units or partial hospitalization units where services are reimbursed through Medicare. With Medicare reimbursement, documentation is similar to inpatient Medicare requirements but the types of intervention covered include psychiatric occupational therapy services as well as self-care interventions (Lopes, 2000).

Psychosocial interventions are at the very the root of occupational therapy and are still fundamental to occupational therapy practice as a whole. From its inception to the present, occupational therapy practice has been wholistic and client-centered, "committed to assisting individuals and groups engage in occupation to achieve and maintain full participation in society" (AOTA, 2004b, p. 670). Whether on a rehabilitation unit or in mental health, the attention to the psychosocial aspects of a client's life of is critical to the ability to resume engagement in meaningful areas of occupation (Kannenberg & Greene, 2003). Client-centered OT means focusing on the client rather than the illness, and creating an environment of acceptance and support that will sustain valued occupational roles (Kannenberg & Greene, 2003). Nowhere is this more important than in psychosocial practice settings, where clients come to us with serious disruptions in their abilities to take part in meaningful occupations.

Initial Evaluation Reports

Initial evaluation reports may reflect the disciplines included in activity therapy rather than each discipline, thus losing some of the professional identity of occupational therapy. Having an "activities" or adjunctive therapy department rather than an occupational therapy department is cost-effective for a facility that bundles therapy into the room rate rather than billing separately for individual therapies. Even so, it is important to do a good occupational profile from which to plan interventions.

All areas of occupation may be affected by major mental illness (Dicke, 2000; Teske, 2000). The occupational profile will highlight the areas of occupation that are dysfunctional or interrupted and provide information about the context(s) to which the client will return.

Intervention Plans

Intervention plans in mental health are usually multidisciplinary. The "therapeutic milieu," or the total environment of the setting, is often considered to be critical in caring for clients who have mental illnesses. The individualized treatment plan (ITP) in a mental health setting is a contract for change between the client and the treatment team. Ideally, after each individual discipline assesses the client's needs and strengths, the team meets to formulate a list of the problems to be addressed. From this problem list, each individual discipline suggests goals, objectives, and interventions for treatment within that discipline. All goals, objectives, and interventions for each discipline involved in the patient or client's care are written into one comprehensive plan. Major problems or concerns identified in the evaluation are documented on the ITP. The client is a participant in the intervention process, and signs the treatment plan to show agreement with it. These plans are similar to those developed by teams in a rehabilitation setting or school setting but differ in that all clinicians work toward the same goals through different interventions.

Success in writing a multidisciplinary treatment plan depends on:

1. The involvement of the client (and family, if they are a part of the client's present life).
2. The willingness of each member of the treatment team to cooperate in a coordinated effort to effect change.
3. Regular evaluation of the effectiveness of the plan and changes in direction in interventions that have not been effective.

In actual practice, however, the length of stay is sometimes so brief that a client may be discharged before a comprehensive treatment plan can be formalized.

Intervention Strategies

Occupational therapists use a wide variety of interventions in psychosocial settings to promote empowerment and facilitate personal change, including:

- Modification of the environment
- Reintegration into the community
- Motivational interviewing
- Cognitive behavioral approaches

Skills training, such as:

- assertiveness
- problem solving
- basic and instrumental activities of daily living
- self-awareness
- role development
- wellness
- social and interpersonal skills
- leisure skills (AOTA, 2000; Brown, 2003).

Occupational therapy interventions focus on the occupations that are disrupted or that the client would like to pursue in the future. Ideally, the documentation of services provided in psychosocial programs reflects the occupation base of our profession. This means that your documentation should be objective and measurable and focused on your occupational profile and on the client's ability to engage in necessary and valued life activities.

Functional Problem Statements

Functional problem statements in a mental health practice setting are traditionally divided into two parts, as noted in Chapter 3. The problem itself is stated in one or two words, such as "chemical dependence", "noncompliant behavior", or "suicide risk". The behavioral manifestations which follow define the areas of occupation and underlying factors involved.

Problem: Chemical dependence

Behavioral Manifestations: Mark has been using alcohol since age 12 with increasing frequency over the last year, and also admits to using cocaine, "crystal", opium, and marijuana, resulting in a failed marriage, loss of two jobs, and involvement with the criminal justice system.

Problem: Noncompliant behavior

Behavioral Manifestations: Client disobeys foster parents by running away, refusal to follow rules or requests, and engaging in sexual activity, resulting in six foster home placements in the past 4 years.

Problem: Suicide risk

Behavioral Manifestations: During the week prior to admission, the client verbalized suicidal ideation, stating that life was no longer worth living. On the day of admission he purchased a handgun.

Goals and Objectives

Goals and objectives are often interdisciplinary in an inpatient setting, contributing to role diffusion and decreasing professional identity. Each discipline works on the same goals, using its individual treatment strategies. Goals and objectives are often selected from computer programs or provided on preprinted sheets for the problems most commonly treated, as illustrated later in this chapter. Because of short length of stay and the multidisciplinary nature of the plan, discharge goals may not be broken down into short-term goals. In community settings, occupational therapy goals can be related more easily and clearly to areas of occupational engagement.

Interventions

Interventions may be specific to occupational therapy, or may be broader and applicable to activity therapy. The choice of interventions may depend largely upon what treatment groups are being provided by the facility, with the ability to individualize intervention strategies within the groups themselves. Selecting meaningful treatment interventions can be an interesting challenge. For example, most clients may attend communication groups, but within those groups, you will customize the way you choose to increase communication skills for each individual client. With a little experience, you will learn to individualize goals for each client in the group, while still providing for the needs of the group as a whole.

When planning intervention strategies, the client's assets (good verbal skills, intelligence, etc.) will be the tools that the client has to use in overcoming her problems. A "strength" in this context is an ability, a skill, or an interest that the client has used in the past or has the potential for using. Assets can include such things as the client's interests (enjoys playing music), abilities (writes well), relationship skills (has a good relationship with her father), and social support systems (minister keeps in contact). Assets may also be past abilities that the treatment team wants to encourage as treatment progresses (Jane was physically active before she became ill). Some interests (enjoys going to bars on weekends) may not be assets.

Contact and Progress Notes

The use of contact and progress notes may vary by facility. One of the exceptions is geriatric psychiatric inpatient and partial hospitalization units where the clients are insured through Medicare. In these settings, the documentation follows Medicare requirements.

If a client with a mental health diagnosis is seen in home health, the Medicare standards for home health, which require treatment notes for each visit, apply. In a situation where progress notes rather than treatment notes are used, the therapist keeps a log of attendance and makes notes to himself about participation and behaviors that show progress each day, and then compiles these into a progress note in the health record at regular intervals.

When you begin thinking in the language of mental health, terms like "brightened affect" or "less delusional," or "improved mood" begin to enter your vocabulary, and you may be tempted to write in less objective and measurable terms. However, there are observable behavioral manifestations that help you determine that the client's affect is brighter or his mood is improved. Perhaps you are seeing him smile more frequently or initiate conversation more often, or respond to your "hello" by making eye contact. Perhaps she takes less time to get up and dress in the morning or is more easily persuaded to attend OT. These indicators are all measurable, and it is very helpful to the treatment team if you are able to report your observations in measurable and behavioral terms.

The trend toward role diffusion is making it more difficult to document occupational therapy as a service that offers good value for the dollars spent in mental health care. As resources shrink and costs expand, we need to focus on documenting functional changes that are cost-effective and meaningful to both the payer and to the consumer. There are myriad factors that hinder ability to engage in meaningful occupation present in the lives of people who have serious mental illness and chemical dependency. In a situation where so much role diffusion is present, occupational therapists need to be clear about the way our services impact the client's ability to achieve "successful, meaningful, and lasting functional outcomes" (Kannenberg & Greene, 2003).

Critical Care Pathways in Mental Health

As length of stay has shortened for psychiatric diagnoses, some mental health settings have begun using critical care pathways and computer-generated intervention plans for the most common problems seen in that setting. These are time savers and can be customized to the client by adding desired outcomes and treatment interventions specific to the individual client.

Critical care pathways in mental health are multidisciplinary and are conceptually the same as those in rehabilitation. The plan for the client's care for each day for each discipline is preplanned in order to make the most efficient use of staff time during the short length of stay, while still making sure the client's needs are met.

Computer-Generated Plans

In an electronic "mix-and-match" program, the computer provides prompts from which the team or the individual therapist selects the problem statements, goals, objectives, and treatment interventions that will be used for the individual client. When using prepackaged treatment planning sheets, the problems are expressed briefly, e.g., *depressed mood, drug abuse, suicide risk*, and the behavioral manifestations that apply to the individual client are written in.

There is a list of long-term goals, or **outcomes**, such as these:

Client will report the absence of suicidal ideation.
-or-
Client will identify 3 new coping strategies to use when he feels the urge to use drugs.

The treatment team chooses goals for each client who is admitted. All members of the interdisciplinary treatment team work on these goals during the client's hospital stay. On a computer generated form, there is also a list of potential interventions that would also be addressed by the treatment team. Interventions might include such strategies as the following:

- *Evaluate the client.*
- *Encourage client to express emotions.*
- *Teach new coping skills.*
- *Encourage the client to verbalize alternatives to previous coping strategies.*
- *Assist the client to develop a discharge plan that will prevent recurrence.*

Interventions are chosen for use with each client. Each discipline implements the interventions in its own way. In relation to the five intervention strategies listed above, you might:

- Do an occupational profile to determine specific problems in each area of occupation.
- Use OT media to encourage the client to express emotions.
- Use OT groups to teach new coping skills and to help the client to find alternatives to strategies that have not worked well in the past.
- Help the client make a plan for any areas of occupation that were part of the previous problem.

Social work adapts the same treatment interventions to individual and group therapy, and nursing implements the interventions on the unit. In this situation, there are sheets provided for each goal that is commonly used. The interventions are individualized to the client by stating behavioral manifestations of the problem and by adding and deleting outcomes and/or interventions.

An example of such a prepackaged treatment planning sheet for alcohol dependence follows. It is provided only as an example of what might be seen in practice.

Behavioral Health Multidisciplinary Treatment Plan

Problem #:   **Problem Name:** Alcohol dependence   **Date Identified:**
Behavioral Manifestations:

Desired Outcomes	Target Date	Date Achieved
1. Client will verbally acknowledge that alcohol use has been a problem and will state an intent to abstain from alcohol use.		
2. Client will have developed at least three new ways to deal with stress and will have demonstrated use of these.		
3. Client will have an aftercare plan in place.		
4. Client will have established a 5-day period of sobriety and of attending AA meetings daily.		
5.		
6.		

Treatment Interventions	Staff Responsible
1. Evaluation of the client's alcohol intake and use patterns.	
2. Provide individual, group and family therapy.	
3. Education re: the disease model of chemical dependency.	
4. Provide opportunities to express feelings.	
5. Teach coping skills.	
6. Assist client to restructure environmental situations.	
7. Evaluate and teach relationship skills.	
8. Facilitate peer confrontation and feedback.	
9. Introduce social/leisure activities that do not include alcohol.	
10.	
11.	

I agree with this plan

_____
Client's signature

In Chapter 9, we considered treatment interventions for Sarah, a psychiatric client admitted after a suicide attempt. If a treatment team were using computer-generated planning for Sarah's care, the first step would be to go to the computer and pull up some multidisciplinary treatment planning sheets. For Sarah some of the choices might be:

- Suicide attempt
- Poor concentration
- Anger
- Poor self-esteem

On each sheet there would be a place to identify Sarah's behavior in relation to the problem. Following that might be a list of interventions commonly used for that problem, starting with evaluation and ending with discharge planning. Interventions that really do not apply to Sarah would be deleted, and any additional interventions that apply to her uniquely would be added. The groups provided by the facility would be listed as interventions, and you would plan for ways to make the occupational therapy groups offered daily meet Sarah's needs. There would be a list of desired outcomes for each of Sarah's identified problems, with a place to add outcomes specific to Sarah's situation.

Documentation in School-Based Practice

When your caseload consists of children in the public schools, you learn a slightly different language for the same concepts. You now work under a treatment plan called an Individualized Education Plan (IEP) and you write problems, goals, and interventions focused on behaviors and skills the child needs to be successful in school. The IEP is a multidisciplinary plan compiled by therapists, teachers, and parents. Based on an assessment from each discipline, the IEP details the current problems, goals, and interventions for the child in all areas including OT for the current school year. The treatment principles and concepts are basically the same. Only the language is different. That language difference, however, is very important.

- The intervention plan is multidisciplinary, and is called an Individualized Education Plan. The IEP is also specific to treatment of the child's educational and classroom problems and needs.
- Functional problem statements are exclusively problems of engaging in occupation in the educational setting, even though the child may have many deficits in other areas of life.
- Goal statements are written for the duration of the school year, rather than using a time line for each goal. In this setting, goals for the school year are called "objectives." Sometimes the format is slightly different, with a "criteria" added to make the goal specific. It is very important not to set goals for underlying factors in this setting.
- Interventions are specific to the educational setting as well, even though the child may also need treatment for problems in other areas of occupation.

Since an IEP can be quite long, the one provided here has been condensed from its original 26 pages to show aspects which are representative or most pertinent to OT.

Individualized Education Plan

Student: Truman T.   **Date of Birth**: 9/17/92   **Parents**: Linda and Ellis T.
Teacher: Mary Ellen W.   **Case Manager**: Sharon Y.   **IEP Conference Date**: 5/23/05
Annual Review Date: 5/23/06   **Duration of Services**: 1 year
Initial Placement Date: 9/27/98
Service Model:
   Regular education: 100 minutes, initiated 5/24/04   ending 5/24/05
   Special Education: 1550 minutes, initiated 5/24/04   ending 5/24/05
Related Services: Occupational therapy, physical therapy, adaptive PE, special transportation
Placement: Self-contained classroom
Assistive Devices: Glasses   **Physical Education**: Adaptive PE
Special Transition Services Needed: Instruction, related services, daily living skills
Specialized Materials: Easel, bookstand for academic and fine motor activities, enlarged monitor for computer, pencil grip.
Notification of Progress: Parents will be given a copy of the goals and progress 4 times per year with the report card.
Present Level of Performance: Truman has been diagnosed with cerebral palsy (quadriplegic), developmental delays, and visual difficulties. He wears glasses and needs written work enlarged. He has a history of ear infections and has bilateral PE tubes in place. Truman displays low muscle tone, with compensatory fluctuating increased tone upon movement. Fine motor skills include spasticity noted in both arms on passive range of motion. Grip strength has improved, but bilateral tasks remain difficult due to poor lateral trunk control. He requires minimal to moderate assistance to hold his arms in different positions simultaneously. He requires moderate assistance to use scissors. His speech and language skills are commensurate with his intellectual functioning, in the mentally handicapped range of abilities. The WISC II suggests that his general information and verbal reasoning skills are at a 6 year age level. Nonverbal abilities are at about the same level. Truman shows difficulty with visual-spatial abilities, visual-motor integration, gross-motor production, and visual-perceptual processing. Vocabulary is low. He has a relative strength in short-term auditory memory and ability to sequence small bits of information. His ability to perceive patterns and relations is impaired, as is his neuropsychological processing of tactile stimuli. His adaptive behavior is below average. Current level of functioning is the 1.0 - 1.5 grade level. Reading comprehension and spelling ability are age equivalent 6-0, with math computation at an age level of 7-0. Adaptive functioning suggests an age equivalent of approximately 5-0 years. He is able to use a telephone in an emergency, look both ways before crossing the street, and get a drink of water from a tap unassisted. Progress has been made in adaptive functioning, but significant deficits remain in regard to toileting, dressing, functional mobility, and food preparation skills. No significant behavioral difficulties exist either at school or at home. Truman has limited interactions with peers, and limited participation in the regular classroom. He attends technology lab twice a week with a student aide. He works best on a 1-1 basis for 15 to 20 minute intervals in a situation where auditory distractions are limited.

Annual Goal #1:   Truman will show school/homework responsibilities.
Implementer: Special education teacher
Short-Term Objective #1:   Truman will be responsible for homework in different areas of study at least 2 times weekly.
Short-Term Objective #2:   Truman will be responsible for taking notebook home and returning it the following day. Homework assignments consisting of spelling words, reading and math sheets, counting change, and telling time. Worksheets will be listed in this book.
Evaluation Procedure: Observation

Annual Goal #2:   Truman will improve skills in adaptive physical education.
Implementer: Adaptive PE teacher/paraprofessional

Short-Term Objective: *Truman will sit up.*
Evaluation Procedure: *Observation*
Criteria: *Without being reminded for ½ hour*

Annual Goal #3:   *Truman will use computers in the classroom and computer lab.*
Implementer: *Special education teacher/paraprofessionals*
Short-Term Objective: *Truman will use computers with assistance.*
Evaluation Procedure: *Observation*
Criteria: *80% accuracy*

Annual Goal #4:   *Truman will improve math skills.*
Implementer: *Special education teacher*
Objective #1:   *Given a clock dial, Truman will say the time to the 5-minute interval.*
Evaluation Procedure: *Daily work*
Criteria: *80% accuracy 3 of 4 tracking days*

Annual Goal #5:   *Improve fine motor for greater success with classroom related activities*
Implementer: *Occupational therapist*
Short-Term Objective #1:   *Truman will cut 8" using adaptive scissors with minimal assistance to adjust grasp and paper position.*
Evaluation Procedure: *Daily work*
Criteria: *75% accuracy*
Short-Term Objective #2:   *Truman will type 10 spelling words on adaptive computer keyboard using isolated index finger movements.*
Evaluation Procedure: *Daily work*
Criteria: *No more than 2 errors*

Annual Goal #6:   *Increase visual motor skills for greater success in academic work*
Implementer: *Occupational Therapist*
Short-Term Objective: *Truman will demonstrate good attention to task and visual motor skills in order to sort 15 small items.*
Evaluation procedure: *Observation*
Criteria: *Within 90 seconds with minimal verbal cues and 75% accuracy*

Annual Goal #7:   *Truman will exhibit increased functional motor skills in the school environment.*
Implementer: *Physical therapist*
Short-term objective: *Sitting on a box, Truman will lean forward and sit upright picking up objects from the floor.*
Evaluation procedure: *Observation*
Criteria: *8 times with 50% assistance from therapist after 10 consecutive sessions*

Least Restrictive Environment: *Self-contained special education classroom*
Related Services: *Occupational therapy, physical therapy, transportation, assistive technology, language therapy*
Will student be receiving services in school closest to home? ____ *yes* ____*no*
IEP services that cannot be provided in the regular classroom: *Math, reading, written expression, listening comprehension, language, physical therapy, occupational therapy, transition*
Factors for consideration of removal:
   1. **Nature and severity of the disability**:
          Difficulty performing activity of daily living at an age-appropriate level
          Receptive/expressive language skills interfere with communication
          Easily distracted/frequently off task

2. ***Diverse learning style of the student***:
>   *Requires highly structured small-group setting*
>   *Lacks social/behavioral skills for participation in regular classroom*
>   *Requires exposure to experiences not available in regular classroom*
>   *Individualized instruction*
>   *Increased drill/practice to master skills*
>   *Immediate corrective feedback*
>   *Additional time to complete task*
>   *Positive rewards*

3. ***Inability to engage appropriately with other students***:
>   *Requires inordinate amount of teacher time*
>   *Learning styles cannot be addressed in regular classroom*
>   *Expressive language skills inadequate for classroom participation*
>   *Receptive language skills interfere with academic progress*

Occupational Therapy Evaluation/Progress Report

This 13-year-old male has received occupational therapy services throughout his school years with intervention most recently 3 times weekly for 45-minute sessions to work on improving fine motor and visual motor skills. Truman lives with his parents who are very supportive, active in his care, and motivated to see him succeed to his highest potential. He has many adaptations in his home to promote independence and assist caregivers.

Truman presents as friendly, kind, and wanting to please. He apologizes when he is unable to complete what is asked of him, although at times he will complain of being too tired to complete a task. He is very social and gets along with both peers and adults. Due to his cognitive limitations, standard testing would not give valid results. For this reason, observation of functioning has been used.

Fine Motor

Low muscle tone with moderate spasticity noted (B) upon PROM. Elbows are contracted by calcium deposits to -30° (R) and -40° (L). Truman is (R) hand dominant. Grip strength (R) is from 15-20# and (L) from 8-16# in the past year. Truman has difficulty with (B) tasks due to lateral trunk instability which requires use of one hand to stabilize himself. He has a hypersensitive startle reflex which activates when he feels like he is losing his balance. He has been working on disassociating arms so that he can use one for movement while the other is doing a different movement, and requires moderate assistance to do this. He is able to open a soda can after the seal has been broken with extra time given. He requires verbal reminders 75% of the time to use his (L) arm to stabilize an object with one hand while manipulating it with the other. He requires moderate assist for scissors use and requires assistance to stabilize the paper. His arms become stiffened as he recruits all his muscle fibers to hold on to scissors and paper. Despite this, he has made great gains in scissors use over the past year.

Visual Motor/Visual Perception

Truman has severe visual problems and needs adaptive equipment to compensate for his visual deficits, including a large screen monitor and adaptive keyboard with the letters in alphabetical order. For future use, an adapted keyboard with enlarged letters in the regular order is recommended. He is able to use the mouse to move coins on the screen into a narrow slot with 75% accuracy.

Truman has a poor ability to track objects and poor ocular motor control. It is hard to tell what he can see, because he often guesses at responses. He is able to find objects in the classroom and to maneuver his wheelchair around obstacles. He has demonstrated great gains in visual motor paper and pencil skills, progressing from the inability to draw vertical and horizontal lines to the ability to copy circles, squares, and triangles with moderate assistance and dot-to-dot guides. Adapted equipment (vertical slant board and enlarged writing utensils) are needed for writing.

Gross Motor

Overall low tone with compensatory fluctuating increased tone upon movement. Specific exercises are performed daily as a part of adaptive PE.

Sensory Integration
No sensory defensiveness or unusual sensory behaviors.

Self-Help
Functional Mobility: *Able to wheel his chair within school environment with extra time.*
Eating: *He generally chooses finger foods but has demonstrated ability to use utensils with built-up handles.*
Toileting, Dressing (coat), Wheelchair Positioning: *Requires moderate assistance for these tasks. He is very private with his toileting and prefers males to assist him. He often slides forward in his wheelchair and has difficulty sitting upright and righting himself once he has leaned to the side. He would benefit from a wheelchair back that provides some lateral support and a cushion that will decrease the slide forward.*

Summary
Truman has made great gains in fine motor strength and visual motor skills over the past year. Harrington rod placement greatly increased his ability to interact within the school environment. He seems motivated to succeed. Strengths include his supportive family, his motivation, his general good health, and emotional stability. Areas of concern continue to be his muscle weakness with compensatory abnormal movement patterns and visual motor/visual perceptual difficulties. If daily strengthening continues to be provided by school staff, Truman would benefit from OT at a decreased rate to focus on monitoring and training staff to assist him with exercise, visual motor and bilateral coordination tasks.

Recommendations
Continue OT services twice weekly for 45-minute sessions to work on areas of concern listed above. Continue use of adaptive equipment listed above. Begin transitional planning for skills necessary after high school.

Linda E., OTR/L

Documentation in Skilled Nursing Facilities in Long-Term Care

Most clients who receive therapy services in skilled nursing facilities in long-term care settings are covered by Medicare and documentation may be done using specialized Medicare forms.

When a client is first admitted, a multidisciplinary evaluation called the Minimum Data Set (MDS) is used to determine the level of care needed. For ease and efficiency, each discipline may be assigned a specific part of the MDS to complete. Facilities may vary in how ADL sections are divided between occupational therapy and nursing. Clients are then divided into Resource Utilization Groupings (RUGs) according to how much care they need. If this process is done improperly, the client will not be able to get the level of care needed. Also, inaccurate assessments and predictions about rehabilitation potential may result in the facility not being able to be reimbursed for care that is provided beyond what was indicated on the MDS.

The initial assessment for a Medicare client may be recorded on a Medicare 700 form (Figure 11-1), which contains a place for the history, any medical complications that will impact treatment, the reason for referral, and the level of function at the start of care. As you can see in the example that follows, there is very limited space available for recording data. The example that follows shows the information recorded in the amount of space that is available. Medicare no longer requires the use of the 700 form, as long as all the same information is present on the form that the facility chooses to use (Olson, 2004).

Progress notes may done on a Medicare 701 form (Figure 11-2), which provides equally small spaces for the reason(s) for continuing treatment for an additional billing period. If you are using the 701 form you must clarify your goals and document the reason for continuing skilled occupational therapy in this section. The requirement for using the 701 form is also discontinued, as long as all the information on the 701 appears on the form the facility chooses to use (Olson, 2004).

| DEPARTMENT OF HEALTH AND HUMAN SERVICES
HEALTH CARE FINANCING ADMINISTRATION | □**Part A** | □ **Part B** | □**Other**
Specify | FORM APPROVED
OMB NO. 0938-0227 |

PLAN OF TREATMENT FOR OUTPATIENT REHABILITATION
(COMPLETE FOR INITIAL CLAIMS ONLY)

1. PATIENT'S LAST NAME Clearwater	FIRST NAME Mildred	M.I. S.	2. PROVIDER NO. XXXXX	3. HICN XXXXX

4. PROVIDER NAME Sandra Matsuda, OTR	5. MEDICAL RECORD NO. (Optional)	6. ONSET DATE 3/23/05	7. SOC. DATE 5/5/05

8. TYPE: □ PT □ OT □ SLP □ CR □ RT □ PS □ SN □SW	9. PRIMARY DIAGNOSIS *(Pertinent medical DX)* pneumonia, Parkinson's Disease	10. TREATMENT DIAGNOSIS Decrease in function 780.9	11. VISITS FROM SOC.

12. PLAN OF TREATMENT FUNCTIONAL GOALS
GOALS *(Short-Term)*
2 wks: Client will be: 1. SBA in bed mobility with adaptations to use bedside commode. 2. (I) $\bar{c}$ sit ↔ stand transfers to bed and toilet. 3. able to ambulate using walker with SBA for safety ↔ bathroom. 4. propel self in w/c (I) ½ way to dining room. 5. min (A) in dressing.

OUTCOME *(Long-Term)*
6 wks: In order to perform ADLs at home, client will be: 1. (I) in mobility & transfers. 2. (I) in toileting using bedside commode or bathroom. 3. (I) in w/c mobility. 4. (I) in dressing and bathing $\bar{p}$ set-up.

PLAN
ADL retraining

Transfer training

Functional Mobility training

Safety education

13. SIGNATURE *(professional establishing POC including prof. designation)*	14. FREQ/DURATION (e.e. 3/Wk. x 4 Wk.) 5/Wk. x 2 Wk. then 3/Wk. x 4 Wk.
I CERTIFY THE NEED FOR THESE SERVICES FURNISHED UNDER **THIS PLAN OF TREATMENT AND WHILE UNDER MY CARE** □ N/A	17. CERTIFICATION FROM 5/5/05 THROUGH 5/30/05 □ N/A
15. PHYSICIAN'S SIGNATURE	16. DATE
18. ON FILE *(Print/type physician's name)* Dr. M. Feitshans	

20. INITIAL ASSESSMENT *(History, medical complications, level of function at start of care. Reason for referral)*	19. PRIOR HOSPITALIZATION FROM TO □ N/A

Client is 73 y/o/f who lived alone and did accounting work until hospitalized for pneumonia 3/23/99 and transferred to this facility 5/1/99. Client states she wants to move to her daughter's home and be (I) in transfers and mobility as in the past. Medical Hx. and complications include Parkinson's disease and frequent falls. Prior to her illness, client was (I) in bed mobility, ADLs, meal & tax preparations. Client was referred by nursing on 5/5/99 2° to client feeling better and being able to benefit from therapy. Cognition: alert and oriented x3; uses phone to direct family and clients from bed. ADL tasks: Client mod (A) in bathing and dressing due to fatigue from illness and complications of inactivity and Parkinson's Disease. Client feeds self after set-up. Mobility: Client max (A) in bed mobility supine to sit; mod (A) in transfers and requires SBA assistance to ambulate in room using wheeled walker for safety and is propelled in w/c outside her room by staff due to fatigue, balance and ambulation difficulties. AROM is WFL but client is slow to initiate movements. Strength is 4/5 in (B) UEs. Grip strength is 10# on (R), 8# on (L). Client is motivated and rehab potential is excellent for discharge to daughter's home with caregiver and possible home health or meals-on-wheels assistance. Client would benefit from skilled OT instruction in safe use of assistive devices, transfer techniques, and home evaluation before discharge.

21. FUNCTIONAL LEVEL   PROGRESS REPORT   □   CONTINUE SERVICES OR   □ DC SERVICES *(End of billing period)*
22. SERVICE DATES FROM   THROUGH

Figure 11-1. Department of Health and Human Services Health Care Financing Administration Form HCFA-700.

DEPARTMENT OF HEALTH AND HUMAN SERVICES HEALTH CARE FINANCING ADMINISTRATION	☐Part A ☐ Part B ☐Other *Specify*	FORM APPROVED OMB NO. 0938-0227

UPDATED PLAN OF PROGRESS FOR OUTPATIENT REHABILITATION
(Complete for Interim to Discharge Claims. Photocopy of HCFA-700 or 701 is required)

1. PATIENT'S LAST NAME FIRST NAME M.I Clearwater Mildred S.	2. PROVIDER Provident Rehabilitation	3. HICN XXXXX

4. PROVIDER NAME Sandra Matsuda	5. MEDICAL RECORD NO. *(Optional)*	6. ONSET DATE 3/23/99	7. SOC. DATE 5/5/99

8. TYPE: ☐ PT ☐ OT ☐ SLP ☐ CR ☐ RT ☐ PS ☐ SN ☐ SW	9. PRIMARY DIAGNOSIS *(Pertinent medical DX)* pneumonia, Parkinson's Disease	10. TREATMENT DIAGNOSIS 780.9	11. VISITS FROM SOC. 10
	12. FREQ/DURATION (e.g., 3/Wk. x 4 Wk.) 3/Wk. x 4 Wk.		

13. CURRENT PLAN UPDATE, FUNCTIONAL GOALS *(Specify changes to goals and plan)*

GOALS *(Short-Term)*
2 wks: Client will: 1. sit ↔ stand transfers ↔ bed, toilet, and bedside commode (I) ; 2. Manage clothing during dressing, bathing and toileting CGA for balance after set-up; 3. demonstrate safe transfers and mobility with SBA from caregiver during home evaluation.
OUTCOME *(Long-Term)*
4 wks: In order to perform ADLs in her own home, client will be: 1. (I) in bed mobility & transfers; 2. (I) in toileting, dressing, and bathing p̄ set-up; 3. (I) and safe in use of walker and w/c in facility & home.

PLAN

ADL retraining
Functional mobility
Safety education
Home Evaluation
Client/caregiver education

I HAVE REVIEWED THIS PLAN OF TREATMENT AND RECERTIFY A CONTINUING NEED FOR SERVICES. ☐ N/A ☐ DC	14. RECERTIFICATION FROM 6/5/05 THROUGH 6/19/05 ☐ N/A
15. PHYSICIAN'S SIGNATURE	16. DATE	17. ON FILE *(print/type physician's name)* Dr. M. Feitshans

18. REASON(S) FOR CONTINUING TREATMENT THIS BILLING PERIOD *(Clarify goals and necessity for continued skilled care)*

Client has made significant progress in 2 wks. as demonstrated in her ability to sit up in bed and to sit on the side of the bed with CGA using a trapeze bar, a firmer mattress and a small bed rail. Client needs SBA c̄ sit ↔ stand transfers ↔ bed; ambulates using walker c̄ SBA for safety ↔ bathroom. Client propels self in WC (I) in her room but requires staff assistance to go to dining room 2° to fatigue. Demonstrates good awareness of safety precautions by using brakes during transfers. Client progressed from mod to min (A) in dressing and bathing but requires help managing clothing, doing fasteners, and bathing back when standing due to ↓ balance and AROM. Client would benefit from continued ADL retraining, transfer and mobility training using assistive devices, skilled instruction and a home evaluation of mobility and safety issues at home with caregiver assistance. Rehab potential is excellent for discharge to her own apartment in daughter's home in 4 wks.

19. SIGNATURE *(or name of professional, including prof. designation)*	20. DATE	21. ☐CONTINUE SERVICES OR ☐DC SERVICES

22. FUNCTIONAL LEVEL *(at end of billing period - Relate your documentation to functional outcomes and list problems still present)*	
	23. SERVICE DATES FROM THROUGH

FORM HCFA-701 ((11-91)   **Form 2701/3P** BRIGGS, Des Moines, IA 50306 (800)247-2343 PRINTED IN U.S.A.

Figure 11-2. Department of Health and Human Services Health Care Financing Administration Form HCFA-701.

Consultation

Consulting work is another area of occupational therapy practice that may use a slightly different method or language for documentation. Occupational therapists may consult on a wide variety of questions about which they have special expertise. For example, a psychiatric unit which relies on recreational therapists and activity aides for its activity therapy program might ask for an OT consult on a client who has both physical and psychiatric disabilities. A newborn nursery might ask for an occupational therapy consult on a high-risk infant. An occupational therapist may be asked to evaluate a work, home, or school setting to make recommendations regarding safety, adaptations for work simplification, ergonomics, energy conservation, or compliance with ADA standards. An OT consultant might be used to peer review charts for quality improvement monitoring or for reimbursement issues.

A consultant gives a professional assessment of what needs to be done, rather than actually doing it. Two of the most common requests for occupational therapy consultations are for consultation on individual consumers, or for consultation on the context in which the consumer works or resides.

Individual Consumers

A consult on an individual consumer is written in the consumer's health record, just as any OT note would be. In a problem-oriented medical record, the note is written in chronological order in the progress note section in a SOAP format. In a source-oriented record the consult would more likely be written in a different format, and would be found in the section of the record marked "consults." It might be in the form of a letter or memo, or it might be written on some kind of form that the consulting OT uses routinely. The following note documents a consultation provided for a psychiatric client who had positioning needs, and is written in SOAP format so that you can see how that would be done. In Chapter 13, there is an example of a consultation on an individual client done in a different format.

Occupational Therapy Consult

Date: 9/12/05   **Time:** 10:30 AM   Positioning Consultation
Mr. E. was seen at the request of Dr. Andrews to evaluate his positioning needs.

S: Consumer reports that he is not able to find a comfortable position in his wheelchair, and that he is not able to propel it in a straight line due to a drag on one of the wheels.

O: Consumer noted to be leaning to the ⓡ with increased pressure on the ⓡ elbow. Back of wheelchair noted to be hammocking badly. Arm rests do not provide a good position for functional use of arms. Gel cushion in chair seems to be working well as an anti-pressure device but transfers cold to consumer. Upon inspection, ⓛ wheel found to have hairs wound around the axle, and also in need of oiling.

A: Several changes in the wheelchair are needed to increase comfort and functional use:
1. Add an anti-sling insert to the back of the chair to provide a more upright posture.
2. Add a pad to the gel cushion to prevent cold transfer of gel to consumer and also for ease of cleaning in case of incontinence.
3. ⓑ arm bolsters are needed for w/c arm rests to bring consumer's arms closer to midline for ↑ functional use.
4. Clean and oil wheels at axle.

P: The adaptations listed above have been ordered. Consumer to be reevaluated after the wheelchair is repaired and adapted.

Lisa P., OTR/L

Settings in Which the Consumer Works or Resides

In evaluating a client's home or workplace prior to discharge, a SOAP note might also be used. For an example of a home evaluation, see Chapter 13. However if a work setting were evaluated for ergonomic correctness or for ADA compliance as a whole rather than in relation to one specific client, a letter or standardized evaluation form would be more appropriate. The following letter documents a work site evaluation that was done on a consulting basis.

MEMO

To: *Earl R. Young, R.Ph.*
From: *Charlet Quay, OTR/L*
Re: *Computer ergonomics in the pharmacy*
Date: *April 14, 2005*

On the above date a visit was made to the 2nd floor pharmacy in response to your request to perform an ergonomic evaluation of the computer work stations located there. This is in response to complaints of carpal tunnel pain, and neck and shoulder discomfort. The following are my recommendations:

1. Computer keyboards must be positioned low enough so that the shoulders can be relaxed during sustained usage and so that wrists can be maintained in neutral position rather than in extension or flexion. When the wrist is in extension or flexion there is more stress on the median nerve that is compressed in the carpal tunnel and may cause pain.

The best position may be achieved by lowering some of the keyboards and/or angling them so the wrists can be kept neutral. Sometimes keeping the keyboards flat or even inclining them with the far end slightly down may help keep the wrists in neutral position. A wrist rest used in conjunction with the keyboard is helpful to some users.

If an ergonomic keyboard is used to avoid wrist deviations it still must be positioned so the wrists are not either flexed or extended. The correct position for each person will be slightly different since all body builds are different. It will be important for each user to know the correct body mechanics and be able to make some adjustments in the workstation to meet his/her needs.

2. The chair should support the back well while maintaining the trunk in an upright position (not leaning back or forward). Thighs should be supported and the entire foot should be supported while sitting in a chair at a computer station. Foot support may be either the floor or a footrest (flat or angled) as needed to support the feet. The rungs attached to the high stools do not allow adequate foot support and may tend to disrupt back alignment. Adjustable-height chairs are recommended to meet individual needs.

3. The monitor needs to be placed directly in front of the viewer so it is not necessary to maintain a rotated position of the neck and trunk. Several monitors were angled to the side, requiring the user to maintain asymmetrical posture, causing neck and back strain. The height of the monitor should be adjusted so the eyes of the viewer look directly forward onto the upper one-third of the screen. This prevents neck strain which can occur if the viewer is having to look up for sustained periods of time.

4. If the mouse is to be used with any frequency it should be positioned near the keyboard rather than requiring a forward reach. A wrist rest attached to the mouse-pad is preferred to remove stress from the heel of the hand.

5. Ideally it seems that the computer workstations should be lowered from high counters to normal table or desk work-height. Table-top should ideally be 26" from floor and the distance eye to screen should be 26" to 30". However it is possible to manage the existing problems with the correct chairs, footrests, monitor positioning, and keyboard/mouse positioning.

6. Taking a break every 30 minutes to do some active movement and stretching exercises is recommended. A copy of sample exercises was left in the pharmacy.

If you plan to purchase chairs, footrests, etc., it would be best to actually go to an office supply vendor to try out specific pieces of furniture, or arrange to have the items on loan so the potential users can check the fit. I hope this is helpful. Please let me know if I can be of further assistance.

Palliative Care

Occupational therapists who work in hospice settings or in other practice settings where clients have terminal illnesses often provide palliative care rather than rehabilitation. Palliative care provides comfort, relief from symptoms, and quality of life as clients prepare for death. In this situation there is no expectation that the client will make progress in physical functioning. Goals often center around pain control, energy conservation, maintaining independence in areas of occupation that are meaningful to the client, obtaining adaptive equipment, and family/caregiver education. Relaxation, active listening, and complementary and alternative therapies are often used with hospice clients. The note below shows one of the complementary/alternative therapies (Tai Chi) being used to increase relaxation and social participation, maintain activity tolerance, balance, functional mobility and satisfaction with quality of life.

Jean is a 48-year-old woman whose throat cancer was diagnosed late and has now metastasized to the brain. She is a single woman who has devoted her life to her career in one of the health professions. She understands her prognosis, and has entered a home-based hospice program where she receives occupational therapy as a part of her care. Jean wants to maintain her social participation and her independence in basic and instrumental ADL activities as long as possible. She has always been physically active, but many of the physical activities she has enjoyed doing with friends are too strenuous for her limited energy.

S: Client states "I feel so much better after doing Tai Chi with you guys, even on days when I think I'm too tired or just don't feel like I'm able to do anything."

O: Client seen in her home for 45 minutes with 2 friends present to increase social participation, decrease risk of falling, incorporate energy conservation techniques taught last week into everyday tasks. Five minutes of warm-up exercises focused on breath-awareness and relaxation were followed by 15 minutes of modified therapeutic Tai Chi with one 5-minute rest period. Client touched chair back as needed for stability during movements requiring weight shift and balance on one foot. Gentle push hands activity was used to challenge balance and to provide physical contact and social engagement during movement activities. Friends remained for short visit and refreshments on the deck, and plans were made to repeat the activity as tolerated in 1 week. Home instruction sheets and a Tai Chi video with relaxation music were provided for use as desired over the next week.

A: Client's homebound status, decreased balance, and variable energy levels limit her social participation and IADL activities. Her perception of increased energy and activity tolerance following the Tai Chi activity allows her to continue to engage in occupation she values. Using furniture as props allows client to practice weight shifting and balance in a safe environment. Physical contact and social exchange during push hands reduced social isolation and distress of "not being able to do anything." Client would benefit from continued Tai Chi activities to address energy conservation, balance, and safety concerns through breathing and relaxation activities done in a social setting.

P: Client to be seen in her home weekly for 45 minutes or as tolerated for 3 more weeks for instruction in mobility, balance, energy conservation techniques to maintain functional mobility, IADL tasks, and valued role as a friend in a modified home exercise energy conservation program.

Different Formats for Notes

Remember that SOAP is just a format—an organizational structure that may be used for any type of note. An initial evaluation can be written in a SOAP format, as can a treatment or progress note. There are other styles of notes that may be used instead.

Checklists, flow sheets, and other similar forms created by the facility are often used instead of SOAP notes to save time. Forms are an especially popular way to document an initial assessment because they allow quite a lot of information to be communicated with little time spent writing. The evaluation/reevaluation/discharge form presented in Chapter 10 was developed by Capitol Region Medical Center in Jefferson City, Missouri. It is a particularly good example because it covers a lot of areas in a small space without sacrificing the ability to individualize the information. It also documents the areas of occupation before the underlying factors, so that no time is wasted documenting underlying factors that do not impact function. Using the same form for evaluation, reevaluation, and discharge allows the reader to evaluate progress toward goals easily. There is ample space for comments so that the form can easily be individualized.

Narrative notes are not formally organized into sections the way SOAP notes are. Narrative notes may present any information in any order desired. Good narrative notes usually contain the "A" data of the SOAP note. Narrative notes reporting primarily the "A" data are becoming more popular due to time and space constraints.

DAP notes are an adaptation of the SOAP format used in some facilities. In this format, the "D" (data) section contains both the "S" and the "O" information.

BIRP, PIRP, or **SIRP** notes are sometimes used in mental health practice settings. Information in this format is distributed as follows:

B: The behavior exhibited by the client
I: The treatment intervention provided by the therapist
R: The client's response to the intervention provided
P: The therapist's plan for continued treatment, based on the client's response

P: The problem/purpose of the treatment
IRP for intervention, response and plan, as above

S: The situation
IRP for intervention, response, and plan, as above

If you work in a facility that uses one of these formats, you categorize your information slightly differently than you do when you are writing a SOAP note.

Electronic Documentation

As we move through the 21st century, as productivity standards become more stringent, and therapists' time becomes tighter, we are beginning to see more electronic documentation. This is bringing changes to the way we approach the documentation task, as well as to the format in which we write. Before we get to an entirely paperless multi-provider system, however, there are many problems to be solved, including what data are available to whom, who is responsible for maintaining the data, and who may modify it (Abdelhak, Grostick, Hanken, & Jacobs, 2001). The ease of access must be weighed against confidentiality and HIPAA privacy standards. At present, we have a wide variety of niche products, many of which may be useful in occupational therapy practice. There are many software packages available to make our jobs easier and more efficient.

There are packages available to schedule our days as well as to send and receive mail, to compile our occupational profiles and intervention plans, to write our notes, and to remind us when everything is due. Software packages for electronic systems offer us a menu from which to choose the initial evaluations we want to use and for recording the data. Other packages offer us choices of problems, goals, objectives, and possible intervention strategies rather than requiring us to compose these for individual clients. Such software can make our job simpler and save valuable health care dollars. However, there are pitfalls to be avoided in using electronic systems (Abdelhak, et al., 2001).

First, there is a temptation to interact solely with the computer in selecting goals, objectives, and treatment strategies, rather than including the client in the process. This should be avoided, regardless of the extra time involved in setting goals and choosing intervention strategies with the client rather than for her. Effective treatment requires the teamwork of the client and therapist working toward mutually selected and agreed-upon goals.

Second, there needs to be a way to individualize each section of the treatment plan or note. A good program will allow editing options or places for comments so that the documentation can be individualized to the client. Medicare reviewers in the past have not looked favorably on "canned" plans and notes that were selected entirely from menus. One way to make an effective compromise between selecting from a menu and individualizing the statements is to use a "mix-and-match" system in which the menu offers components of the statement and allows the therapist to choose the components appropriate to the individual client. For example, in Chapter 9 we looked at critical care pathways for clients who have many of the same needs, and in Chapter 11 we examined mix-and-match treatment intervention plans in mental health. In some situations it is possible to standardize contact or progress note also. In the note below, the computer supplies the words in bold, and the therapist completes the sentences.

S: When asked, client able to state 3/4 **hip precautions correctly**.

O: *Pt seen bedside for ½ hour* **for** *skilled instruction in following hip precautions during personal ADL tasks.*
ADL: *Client able to dress upper body* Ⓘ *and lower body modified* Ⓘ *using adaptive equipment with 2 verbal cues to remember hip precautions.*
Functional Mobility: *Client supine → sit* Ⓘ*, able to walk to bathroom using wheel walker c̄ verbal cues to avoid external rotation when turning.*
Underlying Factors: *Strength/endurance: Client able to lift 4 pounds using* Ⓑ *UEs. Rest break needed after 5 minutes of light activity.*
Home Program:

A:
ADL: *Ability to remember 3 out of 4 hip precautions when asked and to incorporate 2 of the 4 successfully into his ADL routine shows good progress and good potential to follow hip precautions after discharge.*
Functional Mobility: *Client is distracted when he ambulates to the bathroom, and forgets about external rotation when he is turning his walker to enter a narrow space, resulting in continued safety concerns.*
Underlying Factors: *Overall deconditioning has resulted in weakness and lack of activity tolerance needed to complete ADL routine without several rest breaks. Client continues to make steady gains in strength and activity tolerance and has good potential to meet goal of* Ⓘ *in ADL tasks after discharge.*
Client would benefit from *continued instruction in incorporating hip precautions into daily activities and from a schedule that increases activity tolerance and overall conditioning.*

P: **Client to be seen** *twice daily* **for** *2 more days* **to** *complete skilled instruction using adaptive equipment for dressing; to teach tub, shower, and car transfers; and to instruct caregiver in home program.* **By anticipated discharge** *in 2* **days, client will** *transfer into car following 100% of hip precautions and both client and caregiver will demonstrate correct performance of HEP.*

This program cues the therapist to remember areas that need to be covered in the note and provide the words that must be repeated in every note. There is still opportunity for maximum flexibility in individualizing the documentation. You will note that she did not fill in the blank for home program, since she has not yet taught that program. She could omit that section when printing her note, or she could put "Not yet taught".

Finally, we need to make certain that the client is our main focus, fitting the software to the client needs, rather than fitting the client into the capabilities of the software package.

Chapter 12
MAKING GOOD NOTES EVEN BETTER

Now that you have learned to write effective SOAP notes, it is time to review your work and take your skills up to the next level. We will begin by reviewing problem statements and goals, and then we will review each of the SOAP categories. As we review, you will have an opportunity to refine your skills beyond the basics learned so far.

Problem Statements

As you recall, a problem list is developed from your initial assessment. Problems are defined as areas of occupation that are not within functional limits (WFL) and that you plan to address in treatment. Problem statements need both an underlying factor (performance skill, client factor, contextual limitation, etc.) and a related area of occupation. Remember that the best problem statements give a way of measuring the extent of the problem (such as "needs mod assist"). Also remember that those who use our services are more than an assist level, and we make statements in terms of what the client is **unable to do** or **needs assistance in doing** rather than saying that the client **is** a particular assist level.

Consider the following problem statements. Decide whether each one is written as you have learned to write problem statements. If there is one that is not written in the best possible way, please make suggestions about what it needs. You do not need to rewrite the sentence to "fix" it – just make a note of what it needs.

Mini-Worksheet 12-1

Writing Problem Statements

Pt. unable to dress LE ① *due to trunk instability.*

Child doesn't tolerate very much classroom activity due to ↓ activity tolerance.

Consumer acts out.

WORKSHEET 12-2

Writing Functional and Measurable Goals

You know how to write goals and objectives using the FEAST method to insure that all the necessary components are present.

F: Function (If not embedded in the action)   For what functional gain?
E: Expectation   The client will..?
A: Action   Do what?
S: Specific conditions   Under what conditions?
T: Timeline   By when?

However, writing the components in that order sometimes leads to a very awkward sentence. Try rewriting the following goals in a more logical order, making sure that conditions are present in the goal statement.

Client will pivot while standing with SBA during toilet transfers in 1 day.

Client will be min Ⓐ in dressing, UE and LE in 10 days.

Remember that you learned to deemphasize the treatment media when you were writing your observation. This is also important in writing goal statements. Rewrite the following goal statements to emphasize the changes you would like to see in performance skills and to deemphasize the treatment interventions you are using.

Client will place 8 half-inch screws and washers on a block of wood with holes by next treatment session.

Client will make a clock using the appropriate materials while sitting by anticipated discharge in 1 week.

Client will stay in his chair without reminders and spend at least 30 minutes lacing the leather billfold during the 45-minute craft group session in 2 weeks.

From Borcherding S. *Documentation Manual for Writing SOAP Notes in Occupational Therapy, Second Edition.*
© 2005 SLACK Incorporated

The SOAP Structure

Now we will review what kind of information belongs in each category of a SOAP note, and will build a good SOAP note one category at a time.

Subjective

In this section you report anything significant the client says about his treatment. If the client is unable to speak, report on his nonverbal communication, if any. In the case of a young child, a confused client, or a client who is unable to communicate, you may use what the primary caregiver says.

> *S: Client reported that she bent to the floor to pick up her makeup case this morning.*

Or, if the client is unable to communicate,

> *S: Client's daughter reported that her mother bent to the floor to retrieve a dropped item this morning.*

Objective

In this section you report your observations, either chronologically or in categories. This section begins with a statement of where the client was seen, for how long, and the purpose for the session. It is written from the client's point of view, focusing on the client's response to the treatment provided, and de-emphasizing the treatment media. You should be specific about the assist levels. In this section you are professional and concise in your wording, using only standard abbreviations, and avoiding judging the client. For example:

> *O: Client seen for 45 minutes in dining room with daughter present for skilled instruction in maintaining hip precautions during household management tasks. Client ambulated to dining room SBA for balance. Client retrieved snack from refrigerator and utensils from drawer c̄ SBA for safety. Client required 4 verbal cues to remember hip precautions when stand → sit and when turning with walker. Client able to retrieve items from floor after skilled instruction in using a reacher. Education provided to client and daughter on hip precautions and safety during both basic and instrumental ADL tasks. Daughter stated that she understood and would help her mother remember.*

Assessment

This is your professional opinion about the meaning of what you have just observed. In assessing your data, you will pay special attention to evidence of problems, progress, and rehab potential. The assessment ends with a statement of what the client would benefit from. For example, in assessing the observation above, you might say:

> *A: Client's inability to remember hip precautions during household management tasks without verbal cues puts her at risk for reinjury. Supportive daughter and ability to use adaptive equipment properly after instruction indicate a good potential for reaching stated goals. Client would benefit from further skilled instruction in maintaining hip precautions during ADL tasks, sit ↔ stand, and transitional living skills.*

Plan

Your plan contains a statement of how often and for how long you will be seeing the client, your priorities and goals. For example:

> *P: Continue tx. 3x wk. for 1 wk. to work on incorporating hip precautions into ADL tasks. Within 1 week client will be (I) in IADL tasks following hip precautions 3/3 trials.*

WORKSHEET 12-3
SOAPing Your Note

Indicate beside each of the following statements under which section of the SOAP note you would place it.

_____ *Client supine → sit in bed* ⓘ *.*

_____ *Client moved kitchen items from counter to cabinet* ⓘ *using* Ⓛ *hand.*

_____ *Problems include decreased coordination, strength, sensation, and proprioception in left hand, which create safety risks in home management tasks.*

_____ *Client reports that his fingers are stiff this morning and that he is having trouble handling small items like buttons.*

_____ *Client's ↑ of 15 minutes in activity tolerance for UE activities permits her to prepare a light meal* ⓘ *.*

_____ *Child seen in OT clinic for 1-hour evaluation of hand function.*

_____ *In order to return to work, client will demonstrate an increase of 10# grasp in* Ⓛ *hand by 10/3/05.*

_____ *Decreased proprioception and motor planning limit client's ability to dress upper body.*

_____ *Continue retrograde massage to* Ⓡ *hand for edema control.*

_____ *Client's correct identification of inappropriate positioning 100% of the time would indicate memory WFL.*

_____ *Client reports that she cannot remember hip precautions.*

_____ *Veteran would benefit from further instruction to incorporate total hip precautions into lower body dressing, bathing, and hygiene.*

_____ *Learning was evident by client's ability to improve with repetition.*

_____ *Client does not make eye contact during group session.*

_____ *Client's request to take rest breaks demonstrates knowledge of her limitations in endurance.*

_____ *Client wrote bank check for correct amount to pay electric bill with 2 verbal cues.*

From Borcherding S. *Documentation Manual for Writing SOAP Notes in Occupational Therapy, Second Edition.*
© 2005 SLACK Incorporated

_____ *3+ muscle grade of extension in* ⓡ *wrist extensors this week shows good progress toward goals.*

_____ *Client completed weight shifts of trunk x10 in each of anterior, posterior, left and right lateral directions in preparation for standing to perform home management tasks.*

_____ *Unkempt appearance in mock interview situation indicates poor judgment and self-concept.*

WORKSHEET 12-4

Writing the "S"—Subjective

Remember that the "S" or subjective section of your note contains the client's perception of the situation. Sometimes inexperienced therapists simply list anything important the client had to say about his condition. In the example below, all the information is relevant, but does not form a coherent whole. This is not wrong, and it is better than reporting irrelevant data. But it is less skillful than reporting an organized and coherent summary of what the client had to say. Most of this client's comments have to do with transfers.

In the space below, write a more concise version of this "S", remembering to leave yourself out.

> *Client told OT she has real bad arthritis in her right shoulder and knee.*
> *Client said "It hurts to stand on my leg."*
> *Client stated "It [sliding board] needs to be moved further up on the seat."*
> *When asked if she was ok after the transfer, she said "I'm just tired."*
> *Client stated "I'm through" and requested help to get nearer the bed.*
> *When client transferred to the bed, she said "This is the hardest part."*
> *Client stated she prefers to approach transfers from the affected side.*

S:

From Borcherding S. *Documentation Manual for Writing SOAP Notes in Occupational Therapy, Second Edition.*
© 2005 SLACK Incorporated

Writing the "O": Good Opening Lines

When you first learned to write the "O" section of your note, you learned to show your professional skill in the first sentence. For example, suppose you are seeing a client whose contractures are compromising his positioning. Instead of saying "Client seen for positioning", you might introduce your "O" by saying one of the following:

> *Client seen bedside to educate caregivers on positioning to prevent skin breakdown.*
> *Pt. seen in home to select positioning strategies to improve seated posture for mealtimes.*

In another scenario, suppose you are doing some ambulation with a client as a part of ADL activities. Since this might potentially be seen as a duplication of services with PT, you would need to be careful about the words you used. Instead of saying "Client seen for ambulation", you might say:

> *Client seen to increase dynamic balance and attention to Ⓛ UE for safety when ambulating around kitchen to prepare meals.*

In the following worksheet, you will be given an opening sentence that could be changed to show how your professional skill is needed. Below the "old" opening sentence is information that tells you how the skill of an OT was needed in the treatment session. Please reword the opening sentence to reflect how you bring your skill as an OT to the treatment. Use the three examples above as a guide.

WORKSHEET 12-5

Writing Good Opening Lines

Please rewrite the following opening sentences to show how your skill as an OT is important in this situation.

1. Old opening sentence: *Client seen in room for 45 minutes for morning self-care activities.*
Additional information:
- Client is on total hip precautions which raise safety concerns during mobility (especially safe transfer ↔ toilet). Adaptive equipment is available if needed.

2. Old opening sentence: *Client seen at workshop for 1 hr. to work on job skills.*
Additional information:
- Deficits in sequencing tasks, which ↓ his ability to work Ⓘ.
- Bilateral coordination problems interfere with client completing an essential job function of opening/closing boxes.
- Sensory registration deficits contribute to client's high distractibility during task completion.

3. Old opening sentence: *Client seen bedside for 30 minutes for morning dressing.*
Additional information:
- Deficits include ↓ balance and ↓ bilateral motor control of upper extremities that ↓ ability to safely complete ADL activities and use a manual wheelchair for mobility.

4. Old opening sentence: *Client seen in kitchen for 1 hr. to work on Ⓘ in cooking.*
Additional information:
- Client's problems include decreased dynamic standing balance and inattention of affected UE which raise safety concerns.

From Borcherding S. *Documentation Manual for Writing SOAP Notes in Occupational Therapy, Second Edition.*
© 2005 SLACK Incorporated

Being Specific About Assist Levels

Remember that you also need to be specific about **the part of the task** that required assistance, rather than reporting only the level of assistance needed.

Not specific enough:
Client supine → sit with max Ⓐ , sit → stand mod Ⓐ .

Specific:
Client supine → sit with max Ⓐ to lift body weight, sit → stand with mod Ⓐ for balance and to maintain toe-touch weight bearing precautions.

There is a difference between telling **why** the assist was needed, for example:

*Client needed mod Ⓐ to transfer w/c → bed **due to flaccid left side.***

and **the part of the task** that required assistance, for example:

*Client needed mod Ⓐ **to stand to pivot** when transferring w/c → bed.*

In writing about assist levels in your "O", please specify **what part of the task** required assistance.

Mini-Worksheet 12-6

Which of the following statements are *specific about the part of the task requiring assistance*? Please put a check by those you think are correctly stated.

_____ *Client required max Ⓐ x2 bed → bedside commode and bed → w/c and was dependent for pericare.*

_____ *Child required HOH Ⓐ to stay in the lines when following path with crayon.*

_____ *Client needed mod verbal cues to participate in discussion in life skills group.*

_____ *Resident min Ⓐ to don sock due to pain.*

Writing a Complete and Concise "O"—Objective

In the objective section of your note, you report what you observed while providing treatment for the client. As you gain skill, you become more aware of what to include and what to omit in order to be concise. Below is an observation of a treatment session that is very concise. Read it and spend a few minutes deciding what it needs to make it better before reading on.

> *Client was seen in room for further ADL training. Client participated in ADLs and transfer activities.*
> ### *ADL*
> *Client donned robe Ⓘ with set-up.*
> *Client donned/doffed socks Ⓘ with set-up.*
> ### *Mobility*
> *Bed → chair with CGA.*
> *Supine → sit Ⓘ.*

This note does not have enough information. It is *too* concise. There needs to be some indication that skilled occupational therapy was provided. You could start with an opening sentence that shows why your skill as an OT is needed in this situation. As it stands, it is apparent that someone observed the client dress and transfer and recorded assist levels, but a rehabilitation aide or nursing staff could have done this.

Second, the time required to do the activities documented in this note could be very short. If this is an hour treatment session, what else was done? If the client was slow to do the things recorded above, what caused so few activities to take so long? Is there a cognitive problem? Is there a coordination, safety, or motor planning problem? Were adapted techniques or adaptive equipment used to allow the client to be independent?

Third, with this client's documented level of independence, there is nothing in this note to justify further skilled occupational therapy. Unless this is the last session that will be provided, there needs to be information provided that will justify continued treatment.

WORKSHEET 12-7
Writing the "O"—Objective

Now it is your turn. Read the observation below. What does this note need to make it better? Rather than rewriting the note to improve it, just write your suggestions in the box below:

Toilet transfers: max Ⓐ

Toileting: min Ⓐ with SBA 2° inability to support self with Ⓛ arm and to dress

UE dressing: min Ⓐ, verbal cues, set-up, Ⓘ in pulling shirt over head

LE dressing: min Ⓐ pants to hips
          max Ⓐ pants to waist
          modified Ⓘ don Ⓛ shoe (elastic shoelaces)
          mod Ⓘ to don Ⓡ shoe

Ⓡ hand status:
          Ⓡ fingers: small spasticity (index finger greatest amount)
          Thumb: CMC joint painful in abd & flex.
          Ⓡ wrist: flaccid

This note needs:
1.

2.

3.

4.

Writing Effective Assessment Statements

When OTs are first beginning to write SOAP notes, it is sometimes difficult to decide what is an observation and what is an assessment. Anything you see a client **do** is an observation. Its **meaning** in terms of your client's ability to function in some **area of occupation** is your assessment. Sometimes the difference between an observation and an assessment is one of emphasis. You will assess other things besides performance skills and client factors. Often you will assess progress, potential to meet goals, and the psychosocial components of treatment. Remember that no new information should be introduced in the "A". This is an assessment of the data you have recorded in your observation.

In assessing the underlying factors that are not WFL, you learned a formula that helps you be sure you have placed the emphasis correctly and have included all the necessary components.

Underlying factor	Impact	Ability to engage in occupation

It is not the only correct way to write assessments, but it will help you while you are first learning this skill. To assess an underlying factor that is not WFL, you will do the following:
1. Determine the basic or core deficit (such as ½ AROM or *inability to sequence*).
2. Make the deficit the subject of your sentence to give it the emphasis it needs in this section of your note.
3. Decide whether the area of difficulty you have observed today is an indicator of a broader area of occupation. For example, is the decreased AROM you observed to be causing a problem in grooming also a problem in other basic ADL tasks? Will his inability to balance his checkbook also cause problems with other money management tasks? Do the problems you observed today put his safety at risk?
4. Make certain your assessment statement tells how the problem areas impact the client's ability to engage in meaningful occupation. After each problem you note (i. e., limited AROM, sequencing deficits, unstable balance), ask yourself "So what?" So he is unable to do that—what difference does it make? The answer to your "So what" question is your assessment of the situation.

Next we will consider some examples of how an observation statement would be worded differently than an assessment statement.

For example, suppose you are working with a client who tells you she plans to return home to living alone in her farmhouse. You have worked on teaching her some energy conservation techniques, but she forgets to incorporate these into her morning dressing routine. What is the basic or core problem for this client? Why does it matter?

The following statement is an **observation** of the client's behavior:

> *Pt. was unable to use energy conservation techniques during morning dressing due to memory deficit.*

However, phrased differently, it becomes an assessment of what was observed:

> *Memory deficit interferes with client's ability to retain instructions in compensatory techniques such as energy conservation, which limits her ability to safely perform self-care tasks needed to return to prior Ⓘ living situation.*

Note that in the assessment statement, the OT has identified the basic or core problem as the client's inability to retain instructions she has been given. This might be followed by a recommendation to use memory cues of some kind. Otherwise, why should a payer continue to pay for instruction that will not be remembered? You might also want to consider her safety in living alone if her short-term memory is impaired.

According to the formula, the assessment does not repeat what was observed. Instead it begins with the underlying factor that is a problem, broadens the scope of the performance area to include related tasks, in this case all basic self-care tasks, and answers the question, "So what? Why does this matter in this client's life?"

The following statement is an **observation** of what the OT saw today:

> *Client's problem solving was functional and accurate with verbal prompts.*

An assessment of the situation would sound like this:

> *Client's need for multiple verbal prompts to solve social problems limits his ability to respond appropriately in unstructured social situations and to enter into successful relationships with others. Ability to problem solve with verbal prompting indicates good potential to reach stated goals.*

Note that in the observation statement, there was no area of occupation mentioned. In the assessment statement, you are addressing the areas of occupation that are impacted by his ↓ problem-solving skills.

This statement is an **observation** because it tells what the client did:

> *Client tolerated vestibular and proprioceptive input well as evidenced by his choosing the activity.*

Yes, his choosing the activity is an indication of his tolerance, and that is good clinical reasoning, but there are more important things to **assess**. One is his progress in tolerating input, and the other is the ability to engage in occupation impacted by this progress.

> *Client's choices of activities with proprioceptive and vestibular components indicate progress in sensory tolerance necessary for attention to task in the classroom.*

WORKSHEET 12-8

Differentiating Between Observations and Assessments

Identify which of these statements are observations and which are assessments. Remember that an observation will tell you what the client did. An assessment will tell how the performance component that is a problem impacts a performance area.

_____ *Client is unable to don AFO and shoe* Ⓘ *for ambulation.*

_____ *Inability to don AFO and shoe* Ⓘ *prevent her from ambulating safely around the house to live alone.*

_____ *Decreased sensory tolerance limits the client's attention to task in the classroom.*

_____ *Client requires verbal cues to stay on task due to decreased sensory tolerance.*

_____ *Client was unable to incorporate breathing and energy conservation techniques, requiring several verbal prompts to complete task.*

_____ *Inability to incorporate breathing techniques and energy conservation techniques into basic ADL tasks s̄ verbal prompts limits her ability to live alone* Ⓘ *p̄ discharge.*

The following statements are observations of something the OT saw the client do. Reword them so that they become assessments.

Client demonstrated difficulty with laundry and cooking tasks due to memory and sequencing deficits.

Client unable to complete homemaking tasks or basic self-care activities independently due to decreased endurance and not following hip precautions.

After the use of behavior modification techniques, client displayed courteous behavior for the remainder of the treatment session.

Sweeping Assessment Statements

In the face of a busy schedule and serious time constraints, it is tempting to make concise and sweeping assessment statements, such as:

> **A**: *Poor postural stability interferes with ADL performance. Improvement since last note shows good rehab potential. Client would benefit from continued activities to increase postural stability and ability to do personal ADL tasks.*

> **A**: *Client's fine motor, strength, and coordination prevent him from completing ADLs independently. Client's ability to follow instructions shows good rehab potential. Client would benefit from continued activities to increase strength, coordination, and fine motor skills.*

> **A**: *Deficits in upper body strength, fine motor, and feeding limit Jordan's ability to be Ⓘ in home and classroom activities.*

While these are accurate, they are limited, and would benefit from some elaboration. An elaboration on Jordan's note might read:

> **A**: *Deficits in upper body strength limit Jordan's ability to be Ⓘ in eating, functional mobility, or dressing. Decreased fine motor skills will impede typical classroom activities such as holding a pencil or crayon or manipulating small items, as well as age-appropriate IADL tasks in which Jordan is beginning to show an emerging interest. Jordan would benefit from continued upper body strengthening, reach-grasp-release, and feeding activities to move Jordan more expediently through typical developmental milestones.*

Notice how much more information is contained in the examples below than is contained in the examples above.

> **A**: *Decreased cheek and lip range decreases pressure in mouth needed for swallow, which leads to inadequate swallow reflex. Poor suck and swallow pattern due to decreased oral musculature may lead to inadequate nutritional intake. Decreased head control with upright posture indicates poor head righting skills which will hinder Hannah during feeding. Demonstration of visual tracking in different planes indicates good rehab potential. Hannah would benefit from continued skilled occupational therapy for oral motor stretches, increased head control, increased oral motor skills, and a home program for prone position activities.*

> **A**: *Client's ability to complete simple to complex bilateral eye coordination and visual scanning tasks without verbal cues demonstrates increased skill since last treatment session. Client's static visual scanning skills are progressing well, however, client still shows deficits in visual scanning and bilateral eye coordination skills during dynamic movement. Client's ability to perform left shoulder AROM with decreased pain shows improvement since last treatment session. Client would benefit from further skilled occupational therapy in complex bilateral eye coordination and visual scanning, and increased AROM in left shoulder without pain in order to increase performance during basic ADL and IADL tasks.*

WORKSHEET 12-9

Problems, Progress, and Rehab Potential

After you have written your observation of the treatment session, you assess the meaning of the data you have put in the "O". The assessment is the heart of your note, and shows your clinical reasoning. When you are first learning to write notes, it is helpful to begin by going through your observation data and making a note to yourself of the problems, progress, and rehab potential that you see. For any underlying factors not within functional limits, note the performance areas these factors are likely to impact.

Mr. Y. is a 68-year-old male who had a Ⓛ CVA one week ago. His Ⓡ UE is getting some return, and OT was ordered yesterday. Your colleague who assessed Mr. Y. yesterday is out sick today, and you are beginning treatment with him. Her initial note stated that his activity tolerance was not quite 1 minute and she was not sure how much aphasia was present.

> **O**: *Client seen for 30 min. in OT clinic to work on functional movements of Ⓡ UE, dynamic sitting balance, and cognitive skills. Client needed mod Ⓐ in shifting weight to get to edge of w/c and max verbal cues to use correct posture and shift feet during standing pivot transfer w/c → mat. Client requires max verbal cues to initiate grasp of bag in beanbag activity. Client needs mod Ⓐ in reaching with Ⓡ UE. Client demonstrated ability to complete Ⓡ UE shoulder flexion required to toss bag appropriately 2 feet with max verbal cues. Client demonstrated cognitive understanding of activity with mod verbal cues by stating desired goal to be achieved by accurate aim.*

Problems

Progress/Rehab Potential

Now group these and note how they impact ability to engage in meaningful occupation (e.g., safety concerns or ability to care for self).

From Borcherding S. *Documentation Manual for Writing SOAP Notes in Occupational Therapy, Second Edition.*
© 2005 SLACK Incorporated

WORKSHEET 12-10

The School Note

Now we will try assessing and planning for a school-age child. Remember that treatment in public schools always relates to the child's educational performance.

Jed is a second grader who is receiving occupational therapy in the public schools. He has several problems, including low muscle tone which contributes to his upper body weakness and decreased proximal stability. At the time of the last note, he was able to achieve 70% accuracy (with verbal cues) in letter formation.

S: Child stated, "This is hard!" during a bilateral coordination exercise requiring UE strength and stability.

O: Child seen in school therapy room to work on oculomotor movements, fine motor skills required for handwriting, and upper body strength and stability necessary for dynamic UE function in the classroom.

Visual tracking: Child visually tracked a moving object 4 times Ⓡ → Ⓛ @ 40% accuracy and Ⓛ → Ⓡ @ 20% accuracy. Child demonstrated 20% accuracy of eye convergence 4 times starting 12" from nose and breaking at ~6" from nose.

UE coordination: Child performed bilateral UE coordination activity (zoom ball) at 80% accuracy with hyperextended knees and trunk movement to compensate for upper body weakness.

Handwriting: Child able to write letters P, E, F, D, M, N, and R from memory with 90% accuracy and 75% accuracy for staying in line boundaries with min. verbal cues.

What problems, progress, potential do you see in this note?

Write your assessment and plan below.

   A:

   P:

WORKSHEET 12-11

Mr. S.'s Communication Skills

Mr. S. is a 35-year-old male who is in a maximum security unit in a state psychiatric facility. He has criminal charges against him for a violent crime, but was sent to the state mental institution rather than to prison. His current diagnosis is schizophrenia, r/o personality disorder. He was seen today is assertion group.

S: Mr. S. stated that he knows what assertion is, but states "manipulation and aggression have always worked better for me." When asked to explain assertion, Mr. S. stated "the problem with that is the sugar and fruit in the cake."

O: Mr. S. was seen in assertion group for skilled instruction and role play activities to improve assertion and effective self-expression skills. Mr. S. was on time to the group, neatly dressed with hair combed. He was unable to correctly define assertion, and did not respond to any of the three role-play activities, either by taking a role or by offering suggestions to others. During the role-play, Mr. S. placed his head down and closed his eyes. Following the session, Mr. S. quickly left the room.

What problems, progress, and/or rehab potential do you see?

Write your assessment and plan below:
  A:

  P:

A Note That Needs Revision: Lindy's Desensitization

The following note will help you apply the principles found earlier in this chapter. As you read each section of the note, consider what it needs to make it better. In the next exercise, you will be assessing a note in this same manner.

Lindy is a preschool child who is being seen in occupational therapy twice each week to increase her tolerance for sensory input.

> **S**: *Grandma came in with child and stated Lindy was "excited this morning to come see you girls." She also commented that Lindy tolerated a few seconds of teeth brushing this morning. Throughout the session, Lindy stated several times "wipe my hands" or "wipe my arms" when foam got on it for too long. She also cried out and yelled "stop" when she had enough of the oral ranging exercise.*

Revisions: First sentence is irrelevant unless child usually resists attending. Probably the fact that grandmother came is irrelevant, since we have her report. This "S" could be more concise, as follows:

> *Grandmother reports that Lindy now tolerates a few seconds of teeth brushing. Lindy asked for her hands/arms to be wiped off and asked for the oral ranging exercises to be stopped when her tolerance had been reached.*

> **O**: *Child was seen in the clinic to decrease oral defensiveness to be able to begin tasting certain foods and work on self-feeding.*

> **Proprioception/Deep Pressure**: *The therapist began the session with a variety of proprioception and deep pressure activities to allow Lindy to have a better sense of her position in space. Lindy chose to bounce on the big therapy ball first, needing contact guard assist. Lindy then began jumping and sliding which added in a vestibular element. These activities prepped her to engage attentively to the remainder of the session.*

> **Sensory**: *The therapist presented Lindy with foam, water, and foam stick-ups to play with. Lindy was hesitant to play with or touch any of the objects, but after prompting Lindy actually touched the foam but immediately wanted her hands wiped off. Touching this texture is the beginning of a desensitization process that will assist her to be more tolerant of different textures for the purpose of feeding and hygiene.*

> **Oral Motor**: *The therapist introduced the idea of Lindy feeding the babies food in hopes of imitation. However, when Lindy put the spoon to her own mouth, she began spitting. The therapist followed up this activity with completing oral resistive exercises of elongating and protruding the lips and well as stretching the cheek muscles. The intention is to increase length and range for speech and feeding. Lindy had an adverse reaction to this.*

Revisions:
- Delete what the therapist did and reword to focus on the client.
- Deemphasize the media in the first category and talk about the purpose. Keep this brief, since it is only prep for the sensory and oral-motor work, or make it part of the introduction.
- In the introductory statement, talk about sensory as well as oral motor.
- Make the note more concise.
- Avoid mixing "A" material into the observation.

- When talking about desensitizing, tell how much the client could tolerate, in order to measure progress.

   Child seen in clinic to decrease oral and sensory defensiveness in preparation for accepting a wider range textures on skin and in mouth. Child tolerated 10 minutes of proprioception/ deep pressure and vestibular input in preparation for engaging her attention in the therapy activities.

   Sensory: *Child presented with foam, water, and foam stick-ups to desensitize her to textures used in feeding/hygiene, but was hesitant to touch any of the objects. After prompting, child touched the foam, but immediately wanted it wiped off.*

   Oral-Motor: *Child fed the "babies" as an intro to self-feeding. When putting the spoon to her own mouth, child began spitting. Oral resistive activities used to elongate and protrude the lips and stretch the cheek muscles for speech and feeding. Child tolerated 45 seconds before shouting "stop!"*

   A: *Child has increased tolerance for proprioception activities which has led to an increased ability for her to concentrate on one activity at a time. However, her unwillingness to engage in sensory activities with wet and semi-wet media is still a concern in relation to eating. Hopefully with continued desensitization and oral resistive exercise Lindy will have decreased tactile/oral defensiveness.*

Revision:
- We do not see any indication of ability to concentrate on one activity at a time. This is not a problem with the "A", but a change that is needed in the "O" so that we will be able to assess it in the "A".
- The second sentence is good with a little revision. It is a "sweeping assessment statement" and covers a lot of material. Is there more that could be said about the session than this? Are there other problems? What about the problem with tolerating the oral resistive exercises? Is there any progress?
- The third sentence needs to be changed to what she would benefit from, rather than what the therapist hopes.

   A: *Increased tolerance (from 8 to 10 minutes) of proprioceptive activities has resulted in an increased ability to concentrate on one activity at a time. Ability to tolerate 45 seconds of oral resistive activities, willingness to bring the spoon to her mouth, and tolerance for a few seconds of tooth brushing also show progress. Child's reluctance to engage in sensory activities with wet or semi-wet media still present a problem with eating and hygiene. Client would benefit from continued desensitization and oral resistive exercises to decrease tactile defensiveness.*

   P: *Child will continue to be seen 2x wk. for ½ hour per session to increase tolerance of certain sensory media as well as to decrease oral defensiveness. Grandmother will be given education on ways to have Lindy engage in this sort of play at home also. By reevaluation in 3 months, child will be able to tolerate at least 3 types of textures of food, as well as having increased oral range.*

Revisions: No revisions to the plan are needed.

WORKSHEET 12-12
The "Almost" Note

Now it is your turn. This note is **almost** good enough. In fact, it seems quite good on the surface, but has major flaws in organization and clinical reasoning. Mrs. Brown is a 78-year-old female who has had a Ⓛ CVA and has Ⓡ hemiparesis.

What does this note need to make it better? There is no need to try to rewrite the note. For this worksheet, please make suggestions about what needs to be done to this note to increase its effectiveness.

S: Client reports stiffness in Ⓡ hip, but improvement from previous pain. She states a preference for transferring to her left. Client states that she is willing to do "whatever it takes to get out of the hospital."

O: Client seen in room for work on dressing and functional mobility.
Transfer: Client SBA for standing pivot transfer bed → w/c to the left.
Client min Ⓐ with transfers w/c → toilet using grab bar.
Mobility: Client SBA with VCs to flex trunk when rolling from supine to Ⓡ side.
Client SBA supine → sit; min Ⓐ sit → stand.
Client Ⓘ in w/c mobility.
Dressing: Client Ⓘ in donning shirt.
Client min Ⓐ with VCs to don bra while standing.
Client Ⓘ in donning socks and shoes.
Client min Ⓐ with walker and VC in donning underwear and pants.
Client needs set-up for dressing activities.
UE ROM: Ⓛ UE - WFL
Ⓡ UE: ↓ range in proximal shoulder flexion.
Static standing: Client CGA with walker Ⓑ UE support.
Dynamic standing: Client SBA with walker for balance.

A: Deficits noted in Ⓡ UE coordination, Ⓑ UE strength, and dynamic standing balance. Client Ⓘ in dressing EOB, but is min Ⓐin dressing when standing with a walker. Ⓛ UE AROM is WFL but Ⓡ UE has deficits noted in shoulder flexion. Client needs SBA in bed mobility when rolling to unaffected side and min Ⓐ in sit → stand 2° ↑ UE strength. Client needs SBA for transfer to unaffected side in pivot transfer bed → w/c and min Ⓐ w/c → toilet. Client would benefit from skilled OT to continue UE strengthening and coordination exercises and to ↑ dynamic standing balance using walker, in order to ↓ Ⓘ in ADLs.

P: Client to be seen b.i.d. for 30-minute sessions to continue to work on dynamic standing balance. Client will require SBA in grooming activities standing sink-side with standard walker within 2 weeks.

Suggestions for Improving the Almost Note:

Conclusion

Congratulations! If you have read all the material presented in this manual and completed all the exercises, you should be able to document your client care to the most rigorous standards. The notes that follow are intended to provide you with examples of well-written notes from a variety of treatment settings. These examples, along with the ones imbedded in the various chapters, should provide you with ideas for documenting some of the more common kinds of treatment sessions. If you work in a setting that is not represented, you are invited to contribute notes to the next edition of this manual.

We invite your comments, criticisms, ideas, and suggestions for ways to make this book better or more useful to instructors, students, and beginning occupational therapists. We also invite you to submit examples of documentation that you consider to be good examples of some particular concept (such as conciseness). We are particularly interested in notes that represent best practice in occupational therapy today.

When submitting a note, please include your name, address, and telephone number, along with your permission to publish the note. Please send your comments, suggestions, or notes to:

Sherry Borcherding, MA, OTR/L
c/o SLACK Incorporated
Professional Book Division
6900 Grove Road
Thorofare, NJ 08086

The page that follows is a summary of everything you have learned about writing SOAP notes in occupational therapy. Pull it out and carry it with you to use as a quick reference guide while you are learning to document.

A Quick Checklist for Evaluating Your Note

Use the following summary chart as a quick reference guide to be sure that your note contains all the essential elements.

☐	**S:** 1. Use something significant the client says about his treatment or condition.

☐
☐
☐
	O:
	1. Begin this section with length of time, where and for what the client was seen.
	2. Report what you see, either chronologically or using categories.
	3. Remember to do the following:
	   Deemphasize the media.
	   Specify what the part of the task the assistance was for.
	   Show skilled OT happening.
	   Leave yourself out.
	   Focus on the client's response.
	   Avoid being judgmental.

☐
 	
☐
 	
☐
	A:
	1. Look at the data in your "O" sentence by sentence, asking yourself what problems, progress, and rehab potential you see.
	2. Ask yourself "So what? Why is this important in the client's life?" For each performance component not within functional limits, identify the impact it will have on a performance area.
	3. End the "A" with "Client would benefit from..."
	   Justify continued skilled OT.
	   Set up the plan.
	   (Be sure the time lines and activities you are putting in your plan match the skilled OT you say your client needs.)

☐ ☐ ☐	**P:** 1. Specify how often the client will be seen and for how long. 2. Tell what you will be working on during that time. 3. End with a LTG or STG, whichever is more appropriate for your client & practice setting.
	Make certain engagement in occupation is integral to the note. Make certain everything goes together. For example, if you talk about inability to dress in the problem list, don't switch to feeding in the goals and showering in the plan. Remember to sign and date your note.

If you have read the text carefully you will know what each item means. For a more complete explanation, refer to the chapter that provides information in detail. There is a brief explanation of SOAP guidelines on the back of this sheet.

S:

Use something significant the client says about his treatment or condition. If there is nothing significant, ask yourself whether you are using your interview skills to elicit the information about how the client sees things.

O:

- Begin this section with length of time, where the client was seen, and for what reason. For example:
  Client seen for 30 minutes bedside for functional mobility.
- Report what you see, either chronologically or using categories.
- Remember to do the following:
- Focus on performance elements and deemphasize the media. For example:
  Client worked on tripod pinch using pegs.
- When giving assist levels, specify the part of the task the assistance was for.
  Client min Ⓐ for correct hand placement during pivot transfer to toilet.
- Show skilled OT happening—make it clear that you were not just a passive observer.
  For example, don't just list all the assist levels and think that is enough.
- Write from the client's point of view, leaving yourself out.
  Client repositioned, rather than *therapist repositioned the client*.
- Focus on the client's response, rather than on what you did.
  Client able to don socks using dressing stick after demonstration.
- Avoid being judgmental. For example, say he:
  "...didn't complete the activity." Don't add *"...because he was stubborn."*

A:

- Look at the data in your "O" sentence by sentence, identifying problems, progress, and rehab potential. Ask yourself what each statement means for the client's occupational performance. This is your assessment of the data. For example, if in your "O" you noted that client falls to the left when sitting unsupported, what do you think this means he will be unable to do for himself? For example:
  Client unable to sit EOB unsupported to dress.
- Be sure you have not introduced any new information.
- End the "A" with *"Client would benefit from..."*
- Justify continued skilled OT.
  Client would benefit from skilled instruction in energy conservation techniques as well as continued work on AROM of the UEs, strengthening, and compensatory techniques for performing IADL tasks one handed.
- Set up the plan.
  Be sure the time lines you are putting in your plan match the skilled OT you document that your client needs. For example, if you justify skilled OT by saying only *client would benefit from skilled instruction in energy conservation techniques*, then do not say that you plan to treat him twice a day for 2 weeks. Skilled instruction in energy conservation should take only one session, or at most two sessions.

P:

- Specify frequency and duration of treatment. For example:
  Continue tx. one hour daily for 2 weeks.
- Identify the specific performance areas that will be addressed during that time.
  Client to continue OT one hour daily for 2 weeks for instruction in Ⓘ in bathing, grooming, and hygiene.
- End with a LTG or STG, whichever is more appropriate for your client and the practice setting.
  By the end of the week, client will be able to don socks Ⓘ sitting EOB without losing balance.

Chapter 13
EXAMPLES OF DIFFERENT KINDS OF NOTES

This chapter provides examples of notes from a variety of stages of treatment and from a variety of practice settings. The first group of notes illustrates different stages of the treatment process, while the second set provides examples of single treatment sessions in different practice settings.

Chapter Contents

Examples of Notes for Different Stages of Treatment

Examples of Treatment Notes for Different Kinds of Treatment Sessions

The notes in this section were written by students, faculty, and practicing therapists. The signatures are chosen to make the notes anonymous. You may assume that demographic data not present on a contact note is stamped by addressograph card onto the page.

Initial Evaluation Report

Name: Rebecca B.   **Age**: 80   **Primary Dx**: Fx Ⓛ hip
Secondary Dx: Hypertension
Primary Payment Source: Medicare   **Secondary Payment Source**: none
Admission Date: 5/2/05   **Date of Referral**: 5/3/05
Estimated Length of Stay: 4 days   **Physician**: B. Garrett, M.D.
   Brief Occupational Profile: Ms. B. reports living alone and being Ⓘ in all ADLs prior to admission. She had gone upstairs to use the bathroom since there was none on the first floor. She became lightheaded, fell down the stairs, and broke her hip. She was admitted for a total hip replacement yesterday. Her family lives out of town and cannot stay with her. She wants to return home. Ms. B. has supportive neighbors and lives in a small town where she is retired from her position as a second grade teacher. She lives across the street from the elementary school and is in the habit of visiting with the children and some of their families when school is out each day. She is also active in her church.

Occupational Therapy Note
   Date: 5/3/05   **Time**: 8:30 AM

   S: Client stated that she would like to "get this leg well" and go home to "live a regular life."
   O: Client seen in room for initial evaluation of morning ADL capabilities after Ⓛ THR. Client educated on use of ADL equipment for self-care tasks and adherence to hip precautions. Client demonstrated ability to repeat 2/4 precautions. During ADL evaluation client was observed flexing 8°- 10° beyond 90° and required 4 verbal cues to remain at or below 90° during the 45 minute session. Other 3 hip precautions were followed Ⓘ. Client able to complete sponge bath at sink p̄ set-up for upper body, and used dressing stick with washcloth and verbal cues for lower body. Client partial wt. bearing on Ⓛ leg; required min Ⓐ for balance with sit ↔ stand to bathe back peri area. Client able to complete upper body dressing after set-up. Client able to don underwear and pants over hips using a dressing stick. Client able to don socks using sock aid after set-up with verbal cues. Client able to complete grooming tasks and oral care Ⓘ. Following verbal cues, client demonstrated good problem solving by trying different body positions to perform ADLs while adhering to hip precautions and demonstrated understanding of adaptive aids by utilizing reacher and dressing stick correctly after instruction. Client demonstrated ↑ ADL tolerance as she required four 2-minute rest breaks during dressing tasks. Client then seen in OT clinic for evaluation of client factors:
Ⓑ UE AROM—WFL   Ⓑ UE strength—WFL
UE sensation-intact   Grip strength Ⓡ 47#, Ⓛ 43# (Ⓡ hand dominant)
Tripod pinch Ⓡ 10#, Ⓛ 5#   Lateral pinch Ⓡ 10#; Ⓛ 5#

   A: Client demonstrated good motivation, problem solving skills and understanding of equipment use. Upper body strength and AROM WFL, all of which indicate excellent rehab potential. Although she is able to complete grooming tasks and oral care Ⓘ, client is unsafe to complete lower body dressing and bathing due to ↓ endurance, ↓ balance, and inconsistent compliance with hip precautions. Problem areas include ↓ balance in sit ↔ stand, ↓ ADL activity tolerance, and ↓ safety in ADL tasks. These problem areas negatively impact client's ability to be Ⓘ and safe in ADL tasks. Client would benefit from skilled instruction on hip precautions and use of adaptive equipment with ADL performance, therapeutic activities which facilitate dynamic standing balance and ↑ ADL activity tolerance. Exploration of interim living arrangement or possible continued home visits and home equipment procurement if progress warrants discharge to home.

P: *Client to be seen b.i.d. for 1 hour the next 3 days to ↑ Ⓘ in self-care tasks through instruction on hip precautions and use of adaptive equipment, with tasks to ↑ activity tolerance, and balance activities using reaching patterns while standing.*

LTG: *By anticipated discharge on 5/7/05 client will:*
1. Safely complete lower body dressing and bathing modified Ⓘ utilizing adaptive equipment with 100% adherence to hip precautions.
2. Be Ⓘ and safe in toileting using adaptive equipment (walker & bedside commode).

STG: *By 4th tx. session, client will:*
1. Demonstrate ability to don shoes & socks 100% of time Ⓘ, utilizing adapted techniques & devices with 100% adherence to hip precautions.
2. ↑ ADL tolerance as demonstrated by no more than one 15-sec. rest break during lower body dressing task of donning slacks.
3. Safely bathe her peri area modified Ⓘ utilizing adaptive techniques and devices with 100% adherence to hip precautions.

By next tx. session client will transfer with SBA sit ↔ stand using bedside commode and manage clothing with no more than 2 verbal cues.

By 2nd tx. session client will be Ⓘ in sit ↔ stand using walker.

By 3rd tx. session client will be assessed for possible continued home visits and home equipment procurement if progress warrants discharge to home.

Kim N., OTR/L

Intervention Plan

Name: Rebecca B.   **Age**: 80   **Primary Dx**: Left hip fracture/THR
Strengths: UE strength & AROM WFL; intact cognition and motivation to return home

Functional Problems:
Unsafe in ADL tasks due to ↓ compliance with hip precautions following THR, ↑ fatigue,
↓ endurance for ADL tasks requiring frequent rest breaks

Long-Term Goals	Short-Term Goals	Treatment Interventions
By discharge (5/7/05), client will safely complete lower body dressing and bathing utilizing adaptive equipment with 100% adherence to hip precautions.	By 5/5/05 client will: 1. Demonstrate ability to don shoes & socks 100% of time with no verbal cues, utilizing adapted techniques & devices with 100% adherence to hip precautions. 2. ↑ ADL tolerance as demonstrated by no more than one 15 sec. rest break during dressing task of donning slacks. 3. Safely bathe her peri area utilizing adaptive techniques and devices with 100% adherence to hip precautions.	Instruct and have client verbalize 4/4 hip precautions. Instruct in use of adaptive techniques /devices followed by demonstration of use in dressing and bathing activities. Educate client & provide written instructions on energy conservation techniques. Evaluate understanding by her application during ADL tasks; ask about how she performs ADL tasks at home. Instruct in manipulation of clothing and bathing items while standing in walker at sink s̄ violating hip precautions.

Functional Problem: ↓ dynamic balance makes client unsafe during ADL tasks.

Long-Term Goals	Short-Term Goals	Treatment Interventions
By discharge (5/7/05) client will be Ⓘ and safe in toileting using adaptive equipment (walker and bedside commode).	4. Client Ⓘ in sit ↔ stand using walker in 2 tx sessions while observing total hip precautions. 5. Client will transfer with SBA sit ↔ stand using bedside commode and manage clothing with no more than 2 verbal cues by next tx session. 6. Client will be assessed for possible continued home visits and home equipment procurement if progress warrants discharge to home by 3rd tx session.	Instruct client in safe transfer techniques; reinforce compliance with total hip precautions. Provide UE strengthening through reaching and wt. bearing activities at sink and closet for grooming and dressing items and pushing up from chair and bedside commode. Interview client regarding home environment; explore and discuss interim living arrangements or possible equipment use & placement in home; discuss support services needed if discharge home is warranted.

Discharge Plan: To assisted living facility for 3 to 4 wks. until safe in completing all ADL tasks Ⓘ at home with assistance of home health aide if warranted by progress.

Treatment Plan: Cancer

Name: Carol M.   **Age**: 35   **Primary Dx**: Ⓛ mastectomy 2° breast CA

Strengths: Prior to surgery, Carol was in good physical condition and employed full-time. She has some social support from her sister who lives in another state.

Functional Problem:

Carol avoids social outings with friends due to ↓ self-esteem secondary to cosmetic alterations imposed by mastectomy procedure, which precludes her ability to return to work.

Long-Term Goal:

Carol will ↑ social interactions and activity to 6 outings/month within the next month, in preparation for return to work.

Objectives	Interventions
STG: Carol will identify one support group of interest to her within 1 week in order to ↑ willingness to be out in public for work and social activities.	Educate Carol re: available support groups and peer visitation groups, their contact persons, telephone numbers, and ask her whether or not she has made contact.
STG: Carol will attend 1 support group activity within 2 weeks in order to ↑ confidence in social and work situations.	Discuss with Carol's experiences her experiences with the support groups.
STG: Carol will initiate conversation with at least one other support group member during her first visit to the group in order to ↓ negative impact of cosmetic alterations to body image.	Accompany Carol into the community the first time she goes out.
STG: Carol will enroll in a women's exercise program in order to ↑ activity tolerance and positive body image.	Educate Carol re: area exercise groups for post-mastectomy clients.
STG: Carol will identify 5 assets she possesses other than physical in order to ↑ self-esteem and confidence in social and work situations.	Discuss Carol's assets with her, encouraging her to think of as many as she can.

Functional Problem Statement:

Carol is unable to return to work 2° 3/4 AROM, 4-/5 muscle strength, ↓ activity tolerance (fatigues after 1 hr.), and sensory changes.

Long-Term Goal: Carol will return to work part-time by 8/8/05.

Objectives	Interventions
STG: Carol will demonstrate activity tolerance of 2 hours for work tasks within 3 weeks.	Scar massage and myofascial release to incision area along with client education on self-massage.
STG: Carol will demonstrate ↑ of 20° in Ⓛ shoulder flexion in order to be able to reach the items she needs to work.	PROM to Ⓛ shoulder—instruct in self-ranging program.

Active resistive ROM to Ⓛ UE. |
| STG: Carol will demonstrate strength of 5- in Ⓛ shoulder musculature in order to be able to complete repetitive tasks at work. | Resistive strengthening with thera-tubing, weights, and graded functional activities. Work simulation with client education on energy conservation principles.

Provide home exercise program and modify as client progresses. |
| STG: Carol will use correct body mechanics in seated and active work tasks in order to have pain level of <2/10 while working. | Provide education on women's exercise groups.

Educate in ergonomics and posture in order to prevent pain. |
| STG: Carol will observe sensory precautions in work and daily living tasks. | Provide education on safety concerns with sensory loss. |

Progress Note: Hand Therapy Clinic

Occupational Therapy Progress Note
Date: 6/11/05   **Time**: 1:00 PM

S: Client reports pain @ the ulnar styloid with forearm supination. Client reports she is still unable to start her car c̄ her Ⓡ hand but can now use it to turn a doorknob.

O: Client seen in hand clinic for functional range of motion in Ⓡ UE. Moist heat applied to Ⓡ hand and forearm for 10 minutes prior to beginning treatment.
A/PROM measurements for Ⓡ hand and forearm are:

[KEY: flexion/extension; ( ) PROM; - extension lag; + hyperextension]

Ⓡ hand	MP	PIP	DIP
Index	0/90	0/105	0/75
Long	0/90	0/105	0/80
Ring	0/90	0/105	0/80
Small	0/90	-14/105 (0/105)	0/79

Ⓡ Wrist: +45/40 composite (+60/50) composite +45/50 noncomposite
Ⓡ forearm: Supination 62 (78)   pronation 90

Client performed the following exercises c̄ Ⓡ UE:
Isometric forearm supination x10, AAROM supination x5, AROM forearm supination x5. After exercise, client's supination ↑ to 77° AROM. HEP revised to include blue foam for flexion strengthening 2 to 3x day.

A*: Client's gains in DIP flexion AROM since last week is due to ↑ strength of flexors. Active wrist extension ↑ 9° and extension ↑ 5° from last week. ↑ in active pronation is due to ↑ strength while client lost 14° of forearm supination since last week, which appears to be a result of muscle tightness. Client would benefit from continued skilled OT to regain FROM to complete IADLs and for general strengthening.*

P*: Client to be seen 2x wk. for 30-minute sessions. Continue wrist exercises and modify treatment plan to include more supination stretching and strengthening. Client will demonstrate Ⓘ in HEP and sufficient ↑ in Ⓡ forearm supination to start her car c̄ Ⓡ UE in 2 weeks.*

Laurie D., OTR/L

Progress Note: Mental Health

Occupational Therapy Note
Date*: 5/21/05*   **Time***: 1600*

S*: During the first 2 days of admission, Ms. Jones elected not to attend OT group sessions, maintaining that she was too "anxious and overwhelmed."*
O*: Client stayed in her room most of the time for first 2 days despite consistent invitations to attend groups. On this day the client attended a stress management group. Initially she was quiet, but gradually began entering into the activity. She was able to identify specific physical, emotional, and behavioral symptoms that she experiences when feeling overwhelmed or anxious. Ms. Jones stated that she had not been aware of these stress reactions.*
A*: The client is making progress as indicated by her initiating attendance to group, as well as relaxing and opening up socially during the group. Additional progress indicated by recognizing specific symptoms of stress as opposed to relating only general feelings.*
P*: Continue all goals as originally stated. Client to be seen daily for 1 week to provide opportunities for Ms. Jones to learn basic stress management techniques so that she may recognize and control stress reactions when she begins feeling overwhelmed or anxious.*

David L., OTR/L

Transition Plan: Rehab

Date: *2/19/05*   **Time:** *09:00 AM*

S*: Client said "I feel so much better than I did a while back. I feel like I've come a long way."*
O*: Client seen for transition planning from inpatient to skilled nursing setting. Client seen 15/20 tx sessions from SOC. Client illness prevented attending 5 sessions. Client seen for ADL retraining, toileting, functional transfer training, ↑ AROM and strength. Client level of function at transition is as follows:*

Goals:	Initial:	Transition:
Dressing UE Ⓘ	Min Ⓐfor balance	Set-up
LE Ⓘ	Mod Ⓐ for balance	Set-up c̄ CGA for standing to don pants & panties
Bathing: UE Ⓘ	Min Ⓘ	Ⓘ UE
LE Ⓘ	Min Ⓘ	Ⓘ using long handled sponge

Transfers:		
Sit ↔ supine Ⓘ	SBA	SBA
Stand ↔ w/c or toilet Ⓘ	Min Ⓐ	SBA
	CGA c̄ mod verbal cues	
	Shoulder abd-65° (strength 2)	Shoulder abd 90° (strength 3)
AROM-WFL Ⓑ	Shoulder flex-55° (strength 2)	Shoulder flex-60° (strength 3)
	Elbow-0-125 (strength 3-)	Elbow-WFL (strength 4)

A: *Client exhibited an increase in AROM and strength. Client has met bathing and hygiene goals. Dressing and transfer goals partially met. Client continues to make progress and would benefit from further OT intervention to increase UE strength and activity tolerance to perform ADLs Ⓘ and meet all goals.*

P: *Discharged from inpatient occupational therapy 2° change of status from Medicare A → Medicare B. Request physician's orders to reevaluate under Medicare B in SNF. Upon physician's orders, recommend skilled OT intervention 3x week to increase activity tolerance and strength to perform ADLs Ⓘ.*

Carrie C., OTR/L

Discharge Note: SOAP Format

Client: *Ted D.*　　　　　　　　　**Admit Date**: *1/29/05*
OT Order Received: *2/7/05*　　　　**OT Evaluation Completed**: *2/8/05*
Number of Treatments: *5*　　　　　**Discharge Date**: *2/16/05*

S: *Client reports "doing a lot better" and being "less confused" than he was on admission.*

O: *Client initially presented with multiple trauma 2° to MVA. OT evaluation on 2/8/05 indicated client had deficits in short term memory, safety awareness, attention to task, and ADL status. Client seen 30 minutes daily for 5 days for ADL retraining for dressing and grooming and functional mobility. Client and family received skilled instruction in safety precautions in the home. Client's functional status on admit and discharge as follows:*

Goal #	Admit status	Goal	Discharge status
1	Min Ⓐ in grooming	Set-up/supervision	Set-up/supervision
2	CGA in toilet transfers	SBA	SBA
3	Supine → sit with min Ⓐ	SBA	SBA
4	Min Ⓐ UE dressing	Set-up/supervision	Set-up/supervision

A: *All goals achieved due to improved cognitive status, awareness of safety precautions, and skilled instruction in ADLs. Client will need supervision at home 2° remaining cognitive (attention and short-term memory) deficits.*

P: Client discharged to home. Recommend home health OT evaluation for safety in home environment and potential for necessary durable medical equipment. No home exercise program given. No other referrals at time of discharge. OT will follow up in 1 month by phone to check client's functional status in the home.

Laura P., OTR/L

Discharge Note: Facility Format

Name: Marjorie P.   **Health Record #**: 97865
Physician: Fred Dietrich, MD   **Start of Care**: 4/1/05
Room: # 537   **Date of Discharge**: 4/10/05
Primary Dx: Ⓡ CVA   **Secondary Dx**: Arthritis

_X_ Occupational Therapy   __Physical Therapy   __Communicative Disorders

Course of Treatment: Client seen daily for 9 days, 30-minute sessions following CVA to work on ↑ independence in self-care skills, functional mobility, UE strengthening, energy conservation, and activity tolerance.
Status on Discharge: Client reports feeling much better and is ready to go home.

Discharge Status   _Admit status_
Self-care Ⓘ and safe   Self-care mod Ⓐ
Functional mobility Ⓘ and safe   Functional mobility mod Ⓐ
Activity tolerance 7 minutes for ADL tasks   Activity tolerance 10 minutes for ADL tasks

Goals Met: Client has met self-care and functional mobility goals using energy conservation techniques.
Goals Not Met: Activity tolerance goal not met due to client declining last 2 treatment sessions when she learned she was being discharged.

Client/Family Education: Client instructed in and demonstrates understanding of HEP. Handouts given. Client reports having weights at home she can use for continued UE strengthening as instructed in her HEP.

Recommendations: Discharge client to her sister's home due to goals being met. HEP attached. No home health recommended at this time.

Bonnie B., OTR/L

The notes which follow are meant to enlarge the scope of the treatment notes and practice settings found in this manual. These notes were chosen with an eye to their variety.

Contact Note: Acute Care

Occupational Therapy Contact Note
Date: *4/22/05*   **Time:** *15:00*

S: Client nonverbal. Client demonstrated startle response c̄ position change.

O: Client seen bedside to work on initiating and attending to self-care task. When asked to point finger, client required multiple verbal cues and demonstrations, and demonstrated poor response time. Client requires max Ⓐ supine → sit EOB. Client required multiple verbal cues and hand over hand Ⓐ 75% of the time to initiate holding on to washcloth. Client able to bring washcloth to water with 1 verbal cue but required hand over hand Ⓐ to bring washcloth to face. Client attended to looking at self in mirror for ~1 minute. Client required hand over hand Ⓐ to initiate brushing hair. Shoulder AROM limited due to ↓ tone.

A: Overall, client's motor planning, task initiation, and attention during treatment activities continues to be limited. Client would benefit from ranging activities to increase shoulder elevation, as well as further interventions focusing on the skills of initiating and attending to task in order to complete ADL activities.

P: Client to continue OT daily for 20-minute sessions until discharge in ~4 weeks to work on self-care activities and the underlying performance skills and client factors necessary to complete tasks Ⓘ. Client will follow a one-step command in 1 week in order to attend to self-care routine.

Susan S., OTR/L

Contact Note: Cognition

Occupational Therapy Note
Date: *4/5/05*   **Time:** *10:00 AM*

S: Veteran reports feeling fine, but says he does not remember the OTR's name that he has been working with.

O: Veteran seen in OT clinic for cognitive tasks, Ⓡ UE AROM, strengthening and fine motor coordination. Veteran oriented to person, month, year, and place after prompting. He followed two-step commands after max verbal cues and mod physical assist to complete basic self-care tasks. Veteran was unable to grasp and release items with Ⓡ hand. He required mod physical Ⓐ and verbal cues to complete UE AROM used in table top activities.

A: Veteran is not oriented to surroundings at all times, which presents safety concerns. His ↓ cognitive functioning leads to ↓ attention to completion of tasks, specifically dressing, feeding, and bathing. Veteran would benefit from cognitive skills training and safety instruction. Veteran also displays ↓ strength, coordination, and AROM in Ⓡ UE which limits his ability to complete ADL activities. He would benefit from instruction in using Ⓡ UE as an assist as well as from activities to ↑ Ⓡ UE strength, AROM, and coordination to perform self-care activities.

P: Veteran will be seen daily for 4 weeks for 1 hour to improve cognitive skills, ↑ attention to task and safety awareness, and to ↑ Ⓡ UE strength, AROM, and coordination in order to complete self-care tasks. Veteran will attend to task for 10 minutes in order to complete morning grooming within 2 weeks.

Patty N., OTR/L

Consulting Note

This consulting note is not done in a SOAP format, since it is designed to be sent to the school rather than written in the child's health record. This note also provides an example of a note that is done by a student cosigned by the supervising occupational therapist.

Hospital and Rehabilitation Center
Motor Skills Clinic

Name: Brianne Elyse Sample
Date of Evaluation: July 25, 2005
Parents: Irma and Jim Sample
Phone: (555) 888-3988
125 Lewis Street
Columbia, Missouri 65211

Date of Birth: May 20, 2000
Chronological Age: 5 years 2 months

Brianne Elyse Sample is a 5 year 2 month old girl who is being seen today upon request of her family and the UMC Kindergarten Program. Brianne was an active, healthy child until April of 2005 at which time she developed Haemophilus influenzae type-B meningitis. Brianne was hospitalized for 10 days and had a "long recovery" by the family's report. Even though Mr. and Mrs. Sample feel that Brianne has now made a full recovery, they are concerned that this illness slowed her previously fast progress and that she may not be ready for kindergarten this fall. The parents and the UMC Kindergarten Program are requesting an evaluation to assess her readiness for kindergarten.

Assessment Results:

The Fine Motor Section of the Peabody Developmental Motor Scales (PDMS, 1983) was administered to Brianne on July 25, 2005. The PDMS is a standardized norm-referenced evaluation designed to assess fine and gross motor skills in children birth to 83 months of age. Today's evaluation of Brianne (at chronological age 5 years 2 months) reveals:

	PDMS Fine Motor Skills	
	T-Score	DMQ
Total Fine Motor Score:	56	109
Sub-Sections:		
Grasping	73	135
Hand Use	73	135
Eye-Hand Coordination	59	114
Manual Dexterity	53	104

* *T-Scores are based on a mean of 50 and a standard deviation of 10.*
* *DMQ Scores are based on a mean of 100 and a standard deviation of 15.*

Brianne was alert and cooperative throughout the 25-minute evaluation. She exhibited an evolving right hand dominance—utilizing the right upper extremity as the main initiator of activity and the left upper extremity as an assist and stabilizer. Posture, muscle tone, strength, and endurance all appeared to be within normal limits for chronological age. Response to auditory stimuli in the environment was appropriate. The parents do not report any hearing or vision concerns. During the evaluation, the child did not squint, rub eyes, nor exhibit any difficulties with visual regard/tracking.

Summary:

Results of the Fine Motor Section of the Peabody Developmental Motor Scales (given on July 25, 2005) indicate that Brianne Elyse Sample is functioning slightly above the mean in the area of fine motor skills at chronological age 5 years 2 months. Motor coordination and response to environmental stimuli appear to be within normal limits for chronological age. Even though Brianne was recently hospitalized with a serious illness, she currently exhibits adequate fine motor abilities to perform kindergarten activities.

Actions Taken:
Evaluation results were discussed with Brianne's parents who attended the evaluation session today. A copy of this report will be sent to the family and to the UMC Kindergarten Program as requested by the family.

Plan:
Reevaluation upon request.

Truman T. Tiger, OTS ————————————————————
                                        Date:

Christy L.A. Nelson, PhD, OTR/L ————————————————————
                                        Date:

cc: Irma and Jim Sample   dictated: July 25, 2005
      UMC Kindergarten Program   typed: July 27, 2005

Contact Note: Early Intervention

Neonatal Follow-Up Outpatient Clinic
Name: Bobby D.   **Age**: 11 months   **Primary Dx**: r/o developmental delay
Primary Payment Source: Blue Cross   **Secondary Payment Source**: none
Pertinent History: *Bobby is an 11 month 11 day old male child whose adjusted age is 9 months 27 days. He was initially discharged from hospital on August 18, 2004 (Chronologic age 1-04-08; adjusted age 0-01-24). Since discharge, Bobby has been seen twice for medical evaluation at hospital (11-7-04 and 1-18-05). He is being seen today for his first OT developmental evaluation as a part of the Outpatient Neonatal Follow-Up Program. His mother is present at the evaluation.*

Occupational Therapy Note
Date: *3/25/05*   **Time**: *8:30 AM*

> **S**: *Child is not yet old enough to use language to communicate, but makes sounds ("ba, da, ma," etc.) WFL for overall developmental level.*

> **O**: *Today's evaluation reveals:*
> a.   *Atypical patterns of posture and movement (persistent primitive reflexes, presence of tonic reflexes, moderate increase in muscle tone, limited repertoire of movement, and postural asymmetry).*
> b.   *Possible visual difficulties (immature visual tracking and intermittent malalignment (one/both eyes drift inward).*
> c.   *Delayed milestones (child exhibits skills clustering around the 4 to 6 month developmental level).*

> **A**: *These findings indicate that this child is experiencing developmental delay, deviance in the pattern of development, and possible visual difficulties. Bobby would benefit from the following plan of care:*

P: The mother has been informed of the results of the evaluation, and is in agreement with the following plan:

a. Occupational therapy will contact the Neonatal Follow-Up Clinic physician regarding vision concerns.

b. Family is scheduled to return on April 7, 2005 at 9 am to begin joint OT/PT therapy program.

c. Plan to reevaluate developmental status in 3 months just prior to the next Neonatal Follow-Up Clinic appointment.

Christy LeAnn Nelson, OTR/L

Contact Note: Home Evaluation

Occupational Therapy Home Evaluation Report
Date: 2/27/05   **Time:** 3:40 PM

S: Client stated numerous times how nice it was to be home. Client verbalized more in this setting than at the facility.

O: Prior to admission, client lived at home alone with support from family and home health nurse and housekeeping aide and was ① with all ADLs. The following are the results of a home evaluation:

Entry: 2 ½" step, 4" door jam. Uneven grass to step. Concrete broken and no railings present.

Kitchen: 26" area around table in center of kitchen, 27" between snack bar and fridge, 30" high snack bar located on outskirt of kitchen. Little room to maneuver safely. Needs utensils and appliances within reach.

Hallway: 22" from dining room → bedroom with bathroom between inaccessible for walker. Remainder of entries adequate to accommodate walker.

Bathroom: 17" floor to tub top, 18" floor to toilet seat. Bathroom small, but can accommodate wheeled walker.

Other: Throw rugs in all rooms. Chair blocks bedroom access with wheeled walker. End tables block access to living room from dining room with wheeled walker.

A: With the following modifications and recommendations, the home would be safe for client to return to after discharge:

- Remove all throw rugs to decrease falls; remove excess furniture to increase walking area and increase safety.
- Adaptive equipment needed:
- Raised toilet seat with safety rails, shower chair with back support, grab bars, and hand-held shower.
- Add railing to hallway to increase safety without walker.
- Add railing and repair concrete to outside entry.
- Remove kitchen table and utilize snack bar or dining table to increase mobility in kitchen.
- Lower telephone by back door to improve reach.

P: Resident and family will implement the preceding recommendations and changes to allow discharge from facility to return home safely.

Carrie C., OTR/L

Contact Note: Home Health Visit

Occupational Therapy Note
Date: 2/4/05   **Time**: 8:30 AM

S: Client stated that he was "shaky" from his shower earlier in the AM. Client's daughter reported that client showered and dressed with min Ⓐ for balance and coordination to manage fasteners. Client reported that he has been following his HEP.

O: Client seen in his home to assess balance, coordination, level of compliance and Ⓘ c̄ HEP and to introduce new hand strengthening exercises. Client required mod verbal cues to initiate and complete preexisting HEP.

New hand-strengthening exercises added—finger spread with rubber bands of various sizes; intrinsic muscle coordination worksheet, e.g., pen rolling, etc.

Client and daughter participated in discussion about planning treatment activities to compliment client's interests. Gun repair projects and small woodworking activities were suggested for coordination and strength in hands. Client demonstrated good static sitting balance throughout the session, but needed CGA for balance to stand safely from chair.

A: Client demonstrates good understanding of HEP through participation, but required verbal cues to initiate the activity, raising continued concerns about compliance. Client demonstrates ↑ strength c̄ Theraband exercises from 1/29/05 through increased repetitions and decreased fatigue. Progress shown by ability to handle 1" items such as pajama buttons although still has difficulty with smaller items. Rehab potential is excellent. Client would benefit from continued skilled OT to further instruct in energy conservation techniques, safety, and to modify HEP as client continues to progress.

P: Client to be seen 2x wk. for 1 hour sessions to continue work on self-care Ⓘ. Client will demonstrate Ⓘ in showering and buttoning shirt by 3/5/05.

Stacy S., OTR/L

Contact Note: Home Health Mental Health

Name: John W.   **Date**: 2/14/05
Beginning Time: 9:00 AM   **Ending Time**: 10:45 AM   **LOS**: 75 minutes
Goals: 2, 4, and 5

S: John states that having a bank account instead of keeping all his money in cash in an envelope is very confusing to him, and he is never sure any more how much money he has. He also reported some continuing confusion regarding his medication.

O: John was seen in his home for verbal cues to fill his mediset correctly and to review his grocery needs. Skilled instruction provided in meal planning and calculating probable food costs. He was then taken to the bank to withdraw some money, and to a local grocery store to purchase food. At the bank, the teller figured John's account, which confused him. Skilled instruction provided in calculating a bank balance. At the grocery store, John purchased canned fruits and vegetables, ground beef, fresh lettuce, and a loaf of bread. Upon returning home he put the lettuce and meat in the refrigerator independently and consulted his weekly menu planner to determine what he had planned for lunch.

A: John needed only 2 verbal cues to fill his mediset with correct doses of all medications this week as opposed to 4 verbal cues last week. Understanding a bank balance is a new skill for John and he needs continued skilled instruction and opportunities to apply his new knowledge before he is able to manage the account independently. He continues to make progress in choosing healthy foods as evidence by his independent choice of canned fruits and vegetables and the addition of lettuce to his sandwiches. John could benefit from continued skilled instruction in ADL skills such as independent management of medication, food, and money in order to be able to live independently in the community without the support of a professional caregiver.

P: John will continue to be seen weekly in his home and community settings in order to work toward independence in meeting his daily needs. John will fill his mediset independently without verbal cues within 3 weeks in order to decrease the amount of support needed to comply with his medication regimen.

Alan Thomas, OTR/L

Contact Note: Mental Health

Occupational Therapy Note
Date: 4/16/05   **Time:** 4:00 pm

S: Client reported she is currently not volunteering and has not worked for the past 4 years due to her disability status. Regarding volunteering, she says "I need the structure," and further stated that she wants to be productive. Currently, client reports she sleeps "too much," and is having relationship problems.

O: Client was admitted yesterday and attended 4/4 group sessions today. During expressive therapy group, client participated in baking with the rest of the group, but did not eat anything. When each group member identified current emotions, client identified hers as miserable, angry, very anxious, overstimulated, frustrated, frightened, and alienated. During skills group, client identified a possible problem she may encounter upon discharge to be lack of organization, with her "red-flags" being oversleeping and agitation. Client welcomed suggestions from others restructuring her use of time.

A: Client is very perceptive of her emotions and limitations. Her refusal to eat with the group indicates continued appetite disturbance. Client would benefit from information about eating disorders. She would also benefit from continued group participation, with emphasis on increasing self-esteem and time management skills. Client's participation in all 4 group sessions today indicates good rehab potential.

P: Client will continue to attend all daily group sessions while on the acute unit to work on increasing self-esteem and ability to structure her time. Client will demonstrate increased time management skills by naming 5 strategies she will use for gaining control of her daily time by discharge in approximately 4 days.

Nancy B., OTR/L

Contact Note: Pediatric (Preschool Age)

Occupational Therapy Note
Date: *4/7/05*   **Time:** *3:00 pm*

S: Mary said she wanted to play, but when the task was difficult for her, she said, "You do it. You fix it."

O: Mary seen in her home to work on (B) use of UE to ↑ spontaneous use of (L) hand as a functional assist, sitting balance while tailor sitting unsupported, and functional mobility, as a prerequisite to self-care and play skills. Mary was engaged during ~90% of the session.
Bilateral UE Use: *Mary required max (A) to pull shirt over stuffed animal's arms with (R) UE while holding it with (L) UE. She spontaneously used (L) hand to assist with stabilizing animal while pulling sleeve over its arm and shoulder c̄ (R) hand. Mary initiated snapping shirt, but needed max (A) to use (L) hand to stabilize shirt while fastening snaps. (B) hands used to hold animal steady during play.*
Sitting Balance: *Mary requires touch cues from stand → sit in walker and mod physical (A) from side sit → cross legged sit. She demonstrated adequate sitting balance to play for 5 minutes, requiring tactile cues twice to right herself from a lateral tilt.*
A: Mary demonstrated (B) coordination and use of (L) hand as a functional assist ~60% of the time, which is an increase from last week. When she is engrossed in activity, Mary is unable to concentrate on postural support, and needs CGA assist to resume upright posture. She would benefit from continued skilled OT for activities which challenge postural support in order to gain protective responses, body righting, and vestibular integration in order to ↑ her (R) during play.

P: Mary will be seen weekly for 7 weeks to continue strengthening postural support in order to ↑ her (I) in play activities, promote (B) hand use and ↑ use of the (L) hand as a functional assist during ADL and play activities. Mary will be able to maintain upright posture for 10 minutes without lateral tilt within 3 weeks.

Julie S., OTR/L

Contact Note: Public School

Occupational Therapy Note
Date: *4/12/05*   **Time:** *2:30 pm*

S: Heather did not use verbal language to communicate, but did echo words spoken to her.

O: Heather was seen in classroom to work on fine motor skills to prepare for scissors use and improve prehension patterns for writing. After 5 minutes of brushing to decrease tactile sensitivity, Heather worked on palmar pinch and tripod grasp prehension patterns using a "Fruit Loop" bracelet activity for 20 minutes. Heather used tongs (in preparation for scissors use) to pull 15 Fruit Loops out of a cup one at a time. Then using a palmar pinch, she placed each Fruit Loop over a pipe cleaner. Five verbal cues were required for task completion.

A: Heather manipulates tongs well and exhibits a good awareness of positioning of tongs within her hands, which is an indicator that proper scissors use will be attained soon. Good attention to task for entire 25 minutes.

P: Continue prehension activities 3x wk. using a variety of media in 20- to 30-minute intervals until proper scissors use goal is achieved. Heather will be able to cut a piece of 8" x 10" paper in half using adaptive spring scissors (I) 3/3 tries by the end of the school year.

Durwood T., OTR/L

Contact Note: Prosthetic Adaptation

Name: *Daniel P.*   **Med. Rec#:** *87654*   **Client Room:** *455W*
Date: *2/5/05*   **Time:** *3:06 PM*   **Physician:** *Dr. Woodard*

S: *Client appeared pleased with adaptations to prosthetic leg fasteners made this date, stating "this will work."*

O: *Client seen in rehab gym for adaptations necessary to don/doff prosthesis. Client sit ↔ stand ① from w/c while keeping one hand on walker for support. Client positioned prosthetic leg and attempted to fasten straps. Client mod Ⓐ in fastening of straps, ① in undoing of straps to doff prosthesis. Adaptations of prosthetic leg harness completed this date.*

A: *Inability to don prosthesis ① currently limits ① with ambulation/functional toileting. Client would benefit from additional skilled instruction in use of pulley-like fasteners on prosthesis to allow one-handed closure installed this date.*

P: *By anticipated discharge tomorrow, client will don/doff prosthesis ① with added pulley system using strap/loop/Velcro.*

Joanie W., OTR/L

Contact Note: Safety

Occupational Therapy Note
Date: *4/22/05*   **Time:** *10:15 AM*

S: *Client reports ↓ activity tolerance and ↑ shortness of breath with exertion. Client reports feeling ok about asking nursing for Ⓐ c̄ dressing but has urgent incontinence and cannot always wait for Ⓐ to manage O_2 cord to toilet.*

O: *Client seen in room to assess safety during toileting.*
Cognition: *WFL; no deficits*
Functional Mobility: *Client uses walker, has difficulty managing O_2 cord, requires SBA for safety.*
Upper Extremity Strength: *WNL; client fatigues c̄ use of UE.*
ADL: *Client CGA for clothing management c̄ toileting. Mobility during toileting and dressing requires min Ⓐ for O_2 cord management and safety. Client dresses with mod Ⓐ due to ↓ activity tolerance, and needs to stop p̄ 5 minutes dressing activity.*

A: *Client at risk for falls due to inability to manage O_2 cord during functional mobility to toilet. Client would benefit from adaptive equipment and techniques to toilet with ↑ ① as well as instruction in energy conservation techniques and ↑ activity tolerance for ADL tasks.*

P: *Client will be seen 2x/wk. for 1 week in order to ↑ ① and safety in toileting.*

Paige R., OTR/L

Contact Note: Splint

Occupational Therapy Note
Date: *1/21/05*   ***Time:*** *3:00 pm*

S: Mr. J. stated that the pain in his right wrist and thumb was "not as bad as it was 2 weeks ago." He reported that his splint is rubbing a calcium deposit on the dorsum of his hand and that he is not wearing the splint at work during the day. He also reported feeling pain during treatment with movement of the Ⓡ thumb and that ice and iontophoresis ↓ pain.

O: Mr. J. arrived at clinic wearing forearm based thumb spica splint. Upon removal of splint, wrist appeared slightly swollen.
AROM
Wrist flexion ~25%   Wrist extension <25%
Thumb flexion and extension ~25%

Mr. J. tolerated ~3 minutes friction massage over abductor pollicis longus and extensor pollicis brevis tendons. Ice applied for 5 minutes; Mr. J. instructed in using ice at home and at work to ↓ pain by ↓ inflammation of tendons. Splint reformed to eliminate rubbing on dorsum of hand, and Mr. J. instructed in wearing schedule at work. HEP modified and Mr. J. demonstrated new procedures correctly.

A: Swelling ↓ since last tx. session shows good progress. Wrist and thumb AROM are ~50% below functional limits, due to pain upon movement. Limited AROM & pain are causing functional problems in the work environment. Ice and iontophoresis ↓ pain & therefore ↑ functional ability c̄ Ⓡ hand. Splint reconstruction will also contribute to ↓ pain. Mr. J. would benefit from continued skilled OT to ↓ pain, ↑ AROM, ↑ ability to use Ⓡ hand at work.

P: Continue to see Mr. J. 2x wk. for the following:
Ice & iontophoresis to ↓ pain in Ⓡ hand and wrist.
Friction massage to ↓ inflammation and ↑ AROM in Ⓡ wrist and thumb.
Reevaluation of splint for fit and use after reconstruction.
Reevaluation of effectiveness and compliance of HEP.
To achieve goal of ↓ pain in Ⓡ wrist and hand for use in functional activity at work and home. Client will use a screwdriver during work task with <3/10 on pain scale within 2 visits (1 wk.).

Laura P., OTR/L

Contact Note: Wheelchair Evaluation

Occupational Therapy Note
Date: *2/5/05*   **Time:** *1:00 pm*

S: *Client states, "I could get out more with a power wheelchair, like to the shopping center." Client c/o fatigue when ambulating and states that he is not able to drive anymore.*

O: *Client seen in OT clinic for power w/c evaluation. Current manual w/c is narrow, causing sides of client's hips to press armrests into wheels making propulsion difficult. Consult c̄ PT reveals client fatigues and has muscle spasms when ambulating distances of >100 ft. Client measured for power w/c.*
22" wide
18" seat depth 17" knee to floor
18" seat to mid-scapula
w/c features discussed with DME representative. 60° and 90° foot rests tried on manual w/c; client prefers 90° rests for comfort. Joystick control to be placed on Ⓡ armrest 2° hemiparesis. Client requests full armrests to accommodate positioning Ⓛ UE and greater support in transitioning sit → stand. Client able to answer questions re: powered mobility and accessibility in the home and community, and to problem solve for transportation needs such as OATS bus, local accessibility points and terrains and using manual w/c for family visits.

A: *Client has reasonable expectations and understanding for accessibility, mobility, and transportation issues. Potential for using powered w/c is excellent. Client would benefit from skilled instruction in driving w/c using joystick control.*

P: *Client to be seen b.i.d. for 2 days prior to discharge home to work on w/c positioning, adjustment, and driving safely. Client will maneuver powered w/c safely in indoor/outdoor settings by anticipated discharge on in 2 days.*

Desiree M., OTR/L

As occupational therapists and occupational therapy assistants increase their skills in the use of complementary and alternative therapy techniques, questions arise about how to document interventions that may be focused on client factors and that use nontraditional components such as energy work or chakra balancing. Many of these visits are done on a private pay basis, since complementary therapy is often not reimbursable by either public or private insurance. It is best to report objectively on what was said, what was done, what impact the presenting problems have on the client's ability to engage in meaningful occupation, and what the plan is for continued services, just as you would for any service you might provide.

Contact Note: Craniosacral Therapy

Occupational Therapy Note
Date: 2/5/05   **Time:** 4:30 pm

S: Client reports ↓ in functional mobility and ↑ pain since hip replacement surgery. He has adaptive equipment and is able to state 3/3 hip precautions. He reports gains since last visit as follows:
- He was able to sleep 4/7 nights without medication and sleeps longer without waking.
- Headaches occur less often.

O: Client seen in clinic for 1 hour to decrease pain and increase functional mobility needed for work and both personal and instrumental ADL activities. He arrives using forearm crutches in place of the walker he used last week. On evaluation the craniosacral rhythm is asymmetrical, as is the body, with the left side cephalad and the head tilting right. The major restrictions identified are in the pelvis, which is treated first with a series of diaphragm holds and release of the sacrum in supine. With increased symmetry to the pelvis, the Upledger cranial series ending with a long still-point is used to facilitate homeostatic healing activity in the body.

A: Improvement in sleep (decreased need for pain medication and increase in time asleep from 1 to 1½ hours), decrease in headaches, and graduation from walker to forearm crutches all indicate good progress in treatment, as does visual and palpable increase in pelvic symmetry after today's session. Client would benefit from continued work to the pelvis to alleviate cumulative trauma and residual restrictions from recent hip surgery, followed by work to more subtle restrictions that have resulted from a series of previous serious accidents.

P: Client to return in 1 week, at which time reassessment will determine the frequency, duration, and direction of treatment. As soon as pelvic symmetry is improved sufficiently to allow mobility WFL for work and IADL tasks, regional tissue release can be included to increase the mobility of the head and neck which is contributing to the headaches.

Sharon B., OTR/L, CST

References

Abdelhak, M., Grostick, S., Hanken, M. A., & Jacobs, E. (Eds.). (2001). *Health information: Management of a strategic resource*. (2nd ed). Philadelphia: W.B. Saunders.

Accreditation Council for Occupational Therapy Education. (1999). Standards for an accredited educational program for the occupational therapist. *American Journal of Occupational Therapy, 53*, 575-582.

American Occupational Therapy Association. (2000). *Consumer fact sheet: Occupational therapy and mental health*. Retrieved January 5, 2005 from

http://www.aota.org/featured/area6/links/link02ak.asp.

American Occupational Therapy Association. (2002). Occupational therapy practice framework: Domain and process. *American Journal of Occupational Therapy, 56*, 609-639.

American Occupational Therapy Association. (2003). Guidelines for documentation of occupational therapy. *American Journal of Occupational Therapy, 57*, 646-649.

American Occupational Therapy Association. (2004a). Guidelines for supervision, roles, and responsibilities during the delivery of occupational therapy services. *American Journal of Occupational Therapy, 58*, 663-667.

American Occupational Therapy Association. (2004b). Psychosocial aspects of occupational therapy. *American Journal of Occupational Therapy, 58*, 669-672.

American Occupational Therapy Association. (2004c). *The reference manual of the official documents of the American Occupational Therapy Association, Inc.* (10th ed.). Bethesda, MD: Author.

Brown, C. (2003). Interventions for people with serious mental illnesses. In E.B. Crepeau, E.S. Cohn, & B.A. Boyt-Schell (Eds.). *Willard and Spackman's occupational therapy* (10th ed., pp 869-866). Philadelphia: Lippincott Williams & Wilkins.

Contant, E. A. (2003). Coding, compliance, and reimbursement. In M.A. Skurka (Ed.). *Health information management* (pp. 149-174). San Francisco: Jossey-Bass.

Delany, J. V., & Squires, E. (2004). From UT-III to the framework: Making the language work. *OT Practice, 9*, 20-21.

Dicke, A. A. (2002). Mood disorders. In R. Hansen & B. Atchison (Eds.), *Conditions in occupational therapy: Effects on occupational performance* (2nd ed., pp. 75-97). Baltimore: Lippincott Williams & Wilkins.

Gennerman, M. L., (2005). CPT coding: Defining our practice. *OT Practice, 10*, 8.

Holmquist, B. B. (2004, June). Incorporating the occupational therapy practice framework into a mental health practice setting. *Mental Health Special Interest Section Quarterly*, 1-4.

Joint Commission on the Accreditation of Healthcare Organizations (JCAHO). (2004). Questions about goal #2 (communication). Retrieved January 5, 2005 from http:// www.jcaho.org/accredited+organizations/patient+safety/

Kannenberg, K., & Greene, S. (2003). Infusing occupation into practice. *OT Practice, 7*, CE1-CE8.

Kiger, L. S. (2003). Content and structure of the health record. In M. A. Skurka (Ed.), *Health information management* (pp.19-44). San Francisco: Jossey-Bass.

Lloyd, L. S. (2004). Documenting for patients and payers. *OT Practice, 9*, 6.

Lopes, M. (2000). *Medicare guidelines explained for the occupational therapist*. Gaylord, MI: Northern Speech Services.

Mancilla, D. R. (2003).The emergence of electronic patient record systems. In M. A. Skurka (Ed.), *Health information management* (pp. 45-65). San Francisco: Jossey-Bass.

Mandich, A., Miller, L., & Law, M. (2002). Outcomes in evidence-based practice. In M. Law (Ed.), *Evidence-based rehabilitation* (pp. 49-70). Thorofare, NJ: SLACK Incorporated.

Moyers, P. A. (1999). The guide to occupational therapy practice [Special issue]. *American Journal of Occupational Therapy, 53*(3).

Pickett, F. (2003). Health information management and the health care system. In M. A. Skurka (Ed.), *Health information management* (pp. 1-18). San Francisco: Jossey-Bass.

Olson, J. R. (2004). *Coding and billing for therapy and rehabilitation.* Stillwater, MN: Cross Country Seminars.

Sames, K. (2005). *Documenting occupational therapy practice.* Upper Saddle River, NJ: Prentice Hall.

Teske, Y. R. (2002). Schizophrenia. In R. Hansen & B. Atchison (Eds.), *Conditions in occupational therapy: Effects on occupational performance* (2nd ed., pp. 54-74). Baltimore: Lippincott Williams & Wilkins.

Thomas, V. J. (2003). Reimbursement. In G. L. McCormack, E. G. Jaffe, & M. Goodman-Lavey (Eds.), *The Occupational Therapy Manager* (4th ed., pp. 385-417). Bethesda, MD: AOTA Press.

Youngstrom, M. J. (2002a). Introduction to the Occupational Therapy Practice Framework: Domain and Process. *OT Practice, 7,* CE1-CE8.

Youngstrom, M. J. (2002b). The Occupational Therapy Practice Framework: The evolution of our professional language. *American Journal of Occupational Therapy, 56,* 607-608.

United States Department of Health and Human Services. (2003). Summary of the HIPAA privacy rule. Retrieved January 5, 2004 from http// www.hhs.gov/ocr/privacysummary.pdf

World Health Organization. (2001). *International classification of functioning, disability and health* (ICF). Geneva, Switzerland. Author.

Resources

American Occupational Therapy Association at www.AOTA.org

Centers for Medicare and Medicaid Services at www.cms.hhs.gov

Appendix
SUGGESTIONS FOR COMPLETING THE WORKSHEETS

The worksheets in this manual were originally developed for use as in-class exercises. In a classroom situation, students are asked to collaborate on an answer and their collaborative efforts recorded on a flip chart or blackboard. This is a particularly non-threatening way for students to learn new skills, since it allows them to try out ideas and hear the ideas of others as they work toward a correct result. In this situation the instructor can guide their efforts by asking questions to facilitate good clinical reasoning.

In my experience, many of these exercises do not work as well when used as homework assignments. Because there are so many "correct" ways to complete them, they can be grading nightmares. The suggestions offered here as "good" or "correct" are only a few of the many possible correct answers. As you do the exercises with a class, you may collect many more equally "good" answers.

If you are a new therapist using this manual, rather than an instructor, you should be able to work your way through the exercises and check your work against those in this Appendix. Remember that your answer can be different and still be correct, as long as it contains the essential elements. You should not sacrifice your own writing style to be more like someone else's, as long as your information and protocol are essentially correct.

SOAP notes are very difficult to write if there is no treatment session about which to write. Although there are many examples in this manual, there is no substitute for observing or working with actual clients. Only then will you be able to translate your treatment session onto paper in a meaningful way.

Index to Appendix

Chapter 2

Worksheet 2-1: Using Abbreviations

Translate each sentence written with abbreviations into full English phrases or sentences.

Client c/o pain in Ⓡ MCP joint p̄ ~15 min PROM.
Client complained of pain in the right metacarpophalangeal joint after approximately 15 minutes of passive range of motion.

Client w/c → mat c̄ sliding board max Ⓐ x2.
Client transferred from his wheelchair to the mat using a sliding board and maximum assistance of two people.

Pt. OX4.
The client was oriented to person, time, place, and situation.

1° dx. THR 2° dx. COPD & CHF.
Primary diagnosis is total hip replacement. Secondary diagnoses are chronic obstructive pulmonary disease and congestive heart failure.

Shorten these notes using only the standard abbreviations in this chapter.

Client has thirty degrees of passive range of motion in the left distal interphalangeal joint which is within functional limits.

30° PROM in (L) DIP is WFL.

Client is able to put on her socks with standby assistance, but requires moderate assistance with putting on and taking off left shoe.

Client dons socks SBA but requires mod (A) to don & doff (L) shoe.

The client requires contact guard assistance for balance during her morning dressing which she performs while sitting on the edge of her bed.

CGA for balance for AM dressing EOB.

Worksheet 2-2: Additional Practice

Shorten these notes using only the standard abbreviations in this chapter.

The patient was seen bedside for evaluation of activities of daily living. She was able to perform bed mobility exercises with moderate assistance, but needed maximum assistance to put on her adult undergarments. She was able to go from a supine position to a sitting position with minimum assistance and from a sitting position to a standing position with moderate assistance.

Pt. seen bedside for ADL eval. Mod (A) for bed mobility, max (A) to don undergarment.
Supine → sit min (A) and sit → stand mod (A).

The resident came to the occupational therapy clinic via wheelchair escort. The resident was observed to lean to his left. The resident needed verbal cues and minimum assistance in positioning his body in the wheelchair to maintain midline orientation and symmetrical posture. The resident transferred from his wheelchair to the toilet with moderate assistance of one person to help him keep his balance using a standing pivot transfer. He needed verbal cues and visual feedback from a mirror to maintain upright posture.

Resident to OT via w/c escort. Resident leans (L) and needs verbal cues and min physical assist to maintain symmetrical posture in midline. Standing pivot transfer w/c → toilet mod (A) for balance. Verbal cues and feedback using a mirror needed to maintain upright posture.
-or-
Resident to OT via w/c escort. Resident leans (L) and needs verbal cues and visual feedback from mirror to maintain upright symmetrical posture in midline. Standing pivot w/c → toilet mod (A) for balance.

The veteran was seen in his own room seated in a wheelchair for an evaluation of relevant client factors. The veteran's short-term memory was three out of three for immediate recall, one out of three after 1 minute, and zero out of three with verbal cues after 5 minutes. The left upper extremity shoulder flexion was a grade of 4, shoulder extension was a grade of 4, elbow flexion was a grade of 4, elbow extension was a grade of 4, wrist extension was a grade of 4 minus, wrist flexion was a grade of 4 minus, and grip strength was 8 pounds. The left upper extremity light touch is intact. The right upper extremity muscle grades are within functional limits.

Veteran seen in room seated in w/c for eval. of client factors. Short-term memory 3/3 immediate recall, 1/3 after 1 minute, 0/3 c̄ verbal cues after 5 min. (L) shoulder and elbow strength grade 4, wrist strength 4-, grip strength 8#. Light touch intact. (R) UE WFL.

Chapter 3

Worksheet 3-1: Identifying the Underlying Factor

Consumer is unable to sustain employment longer than 2 weeks due to:

Use of inflammatory language at work
Aggressive behaviors on the job
Need for frequent redirection to task
Drug-seeking behaviors at work
Inability to plan and sequence a task
Inattention to social cues and personal hygiene
Arriving late 3 to 4 times weekly following nightly alcohol use
Inability to complete job tasks independently
Lack of reliable daycare

Veteran needs 1½ hours to complete grooming activities due to:

Motor planning deficits
SOB on exertion and need for frequent rest breaks to regain O_2 saturation
<5 minutes activity tolerance before needing rest breaks
Inability to sequence the task
Slowness in locating items needed for grooming 2° low vision
Intention tremors and rigidity 2° Parkinson's Disease
Decreased fine motor manipulation in Ⓛ UE
Muscle weakness and limited AROM in both upper extremities
Inaccessible bathroom
Stiffness and pain from arthritis

Worksheet 3-2: Writing Functional Problem Statements

Without having seen the client in question, it is impossible to know exactly what the correct problem statement would have been. Here are some possible ways that functional problem statements might have been written for the problems given:

1. The client has acquired an injury to his brain. As a result, he is not able to pay attention to task for very long at a time, and is having trouble completing his morning routine. Usually he can pay attention to what he is doing for about 2 minutes, and needs to be re-directed back to the task after that.

> *<3 minute attention span 2° ABI interferes with ability to complete ADL tasks.*
> *-or-*
> *Client able to attend to dressing activity for ~2 minutes 2° ABI.*

2. The child is having trouble in school because she has difficulty staying within the lines when she is writing. She habitually grips her pencil in a gross grasp, although with help (someone's hand placed over hers) she can hold it with her thumb and 2 fingers.

> *Child needs HOH Ⓐ to hold pencil in tripod pinch for writing task at school.*
> *-or-*
> *Inability to maintain tripod pinch unassisted limits child's ability to stay within the lines during writing task at school.*

3. The resident is not very cognitively aware. About 40% of the time she has trouble figuring out what to do first if she has to complete a self-care task, and she doesn't remember what she has just been told.

> *Resident needs mod verbal assistance in ADL tasks due to ↑ ability to sequence steps of task.*
> *-or-*
> *Memory and sequencing problems result in safety concerns during IADL tasks.*

4. Mr. J. has recently sustained a Ⓡ CVA. His Ⓛ upper extremity is flaccid and he forgets it is there. He needs physical and verbal help with ADL tasks about 60% of the time.

> *Client requires max Ⓐ to dress upper body due to flaccid Ⓛ UE and Ⓛ side neglect.*
> *-or-*
> *Client max Ⓐ donning shirt over UE due to Ⓛ side neglect as a result of Ⓡ CVA.*
> *-or-*
> *Client max Ⓐ in feeding due to flaccidity in dominant Ⓛ UE.*
> *-or-*
> *Flaccidity in Ⓛ UE and Ⓛ neglect results in max Ⓐ in grooming and hygiene.*

5. The consumer has had trouble finding a job. His appearance is unkempt and he has a strong body odor, neither of which appear troubling to him.

> *Inattention to personal hygiene interferes with consumer's ability to find employment.*
> *-or-*
> *Consumer has difficulty finding employment due to unkempt appearance and inattention to personal hygiene.*

6. The client is unable to transfer safely w/c ↔ toilet without someone to remind him that he needs to follow his total hip precautions.

> *Client requires SBA w/c ↔ toilet due to unfamiliarity with hip precautions.*
> *-or-*
> *Client SBA c̄ transfer w/c ↔ toilet to follow hip precautions 2° recent THR.*

Chapter 4

Worksheet 4-1: Choosing Goals for Health Necessity

Problem: Client unable to perform sewing due to 2+ strength in Ⓡ hand musculature.
LTG: Client will be able to perform embroidery Ⓘ for 20 minutes within 5 months.
STG: In order to ↑ performance of embroidery, client will be able to use needle continuously for 5 minutes by 11/6/05.

Other Possible Problem Statements

> *Client unable to handle small items needed for grooming due to 2+ strength in Ⓡ hand musculature.*
> *LTG: Client will be able to complete grooming activities Ⓘ within 1 month.*
> *STG: Client will be able to remove lid from toothpaste within 2 weeks.*

> *Client unable to write >3 minutes due to 2+ strength in her Ⓡ hand musculature.*
> *LTG: Client will write for 15 minutes with one rest break within 1 month.*
> *STG: Client will be able to sign first name within 1 week.*

> *Client unable to fasten clothing due to 2+ strength in Ⓡ hand.*
> *LTG: Client will be able to fasten clothing Ⓘ within 3 weeks.*
> *STG: Client will be able to button one 1" button within 1 week.*

Worksheet 4-2: Evaluating Goal Statements

Refer to your FEAST elements to determine which of the following goals has each of the necessary components to be useful in occupational therapy documentation. For each goal that you find to be incomplete or inaccurate in some way, please indicate what it lacks.

1. By the time of discharge in 2 weeks, client will be able to dress himself with min Ⓐ for balance using a sock aid and reacher while sitting in a wheelchair.

This goal has all the necessary components to be useful.

2. Client will tolerate 10 minutes of treatment daily.

This goal lacks a function and a time frame. In addition, the behavior (tolerating treatment) is not useful because it is not something a client needs to do after discharge. This would be better stated as "tolerate 10 minutes of grooming/hygiene activity."

3. Client will demonstrate increased coping skills in order to live at home with her granddaughter within 2 weeks.

This goal lacks specificity, and it needs a condition. "Coping skills" is far too broad. The coping skill(s) in question need to be specified.

4. Client will demonstrate 15 minutes of activity tolerance without rest breaks using Ⓑ UE in order to complete ADL tasks before breakfast each morning.

This goal lacks a time frame, and needs to be turned around to put function first. *Client will be able to complete basic ADL in <15 minutes without rest breaks before breakfast each morning within 2 weeks.*

5. In order to be able to toilet self Ⓘ after discharge, client will demonstrate ability to perform a sliding board transfer w/c → mat within the next week.

This goal has all the necessary components to be useful, but would be even better if the assist level of the transfer were noted (i.e., Ⓘ).

6. OT will teach lower body dressing using a reacher, dressing stick and sock aid within 3 tx. sessions.

This goal lacks a proper actor and behavior.

7. In order to return to living independently, patient will demonstrate ability to balance his checkbook.

This goal lacks a time frame, and would be even better if the assist level for balancing his checkbook were specified (i.e., ability to balance his checkbook Ⓘ).

Worksheet 4-3: Writing Realistic, Functional, Measurable Goals

Without knowing the client, it is impossible to know what the goal would really be. Here are some suggestions.

1. Mary is not able to attend to task for more than a few minutes, which makes IADL activities difficult for her. Since she likes to cook and plans to return to cooking after discharge, you have been working with her in the kitchen. You would like to see her able to attend to task for 10 minutes by the time she is discharged next week. Write a goal to increase Mary's attention span.

Client will attend to a cooking activity >10 minutes without having to be redirected within 3 treatment sessions.

-or-

In order to live ① after discharge, client will demonstrate 10-minute attention span during cooking activity by the end of the 3ʳᵈ treatment session.

2. Now write a goal for Mary to be able to follow directions so that she can read the back of a boxed meal, and eventually a recipe, when she is cooking.

By anticipated discharge in 1 week, client will complete 3-step written directions for cooking a packaged meal c̄ min. assist.
-or-
Client will demonstrate ability to correctly follow a simple recipe within 1 week.

3. Bill is having trouble dressing himself after his stroke. You have been teaching him an over-the-head method for putting on his shirt, and have given him a buttonhook to use. Write a dressing goal for Bill.

Client will be able to don shirt ① using the over-the-head method and a button hook within 2 tx. sessions.
-or-
After skilled instruction, client will be able to dress upper body ① using one handed techniques and adaptive equipment within 1 week.

4. Susan is very weak, and wants to be able to go back to work as a receptionist. She also wants to be able to care for her 4-month-old child. Write a goal to increase her activity tolerance. Discharge is ~2 weeks away.

Client will perform >10 minutes of continuous standing activity in order to be able to bathe her baby by discharge in 2 weeks.
-or-
Within 1 week, client will complete 30 minutes of seated activity without rest breaks in order to return to her job as a receptionist.

5. Sam wants to live independently in the community, but lacks basic money management skills. Write a goal for Sam to improve his money management skills.

Client will demonstrate ability to make change ① from $1.00 correctly 3/3 tries within 2 weeks.
-or-
Client will be able to select ads from the newspaper for an apartment that rents for less than 1/3 of his regular monthly income within the next month.

6. Audrey has become increasingly more depressed over the past several weeks, and was admitted after a suicide attempt. You estimate that you will have her in groups for 1 week. You would like to see her mood change in that week. Write a goal that will indicate an improved mood.

Within 1 week, client will spontaneously follow her daily schedule, as demonstrated by attending at least 3 scheduled activities per day.
-or-
Client will verbalize an interest in at least one future activity within the next 2 days.

Chapter 5

Worksheet 5-1: Writing Concise, Coherent Statements

Client reports using adaptive equipment to don pants and socks while maintaining hip precautions without difficulty. She has no c/o pain with transfers using raised toilet seat. Her daughter now has bathroom equipment in home that was ordered by OT last week.

Worksheet 5-2: Choosing a Subjective Statement

1. Even though the client may have been cooperative, and even though it may have been important in this treatment session, it is an assessment of the situation, and does not belong in the "S" category of the note. The client's social conversation might be important in some situations. However, there is a better choice for this particular note.

2. In this instance, a pending visit by the client's grandson is not really relevant to the treatment session or to how the client sees her progress. It might be important in another situation. For example, if the client were planning to go to live with her grandson after discharge, it might be very relevant, and might be a topic the OT wanted to explore further with the client.

3. Feeling "pretty good" today might be important, because it might show progress or a change in her condition. In this case, however, it is not the best choice.

4. The client's observations about her upper extremity seem most pertinent to this treatment session. Use of the Ⓡ UE is relevant in all aspects of this treatment session.

5. A report of safety concerns by nursing might be relevant to this client's treatment. However, it is not the best choice for the "S" category of this note, for several reasons. A concern by nursing staff should be documented in the nursing notes. The OT should report what she sees, rather than what some other staff member believes. Finally, the subjective section of the SOAP note is used to document the client's views about treatment rather than the staff's views, except in rare instances.

Chapter 6

Worksheet 6-1: Using Categories

Some or all of the following categories might be used to make this note easier to read:
Ⓛ UE use or reach/grasp/release
Feeding
Attention/attention to task/attention span
Splint

Depending on the categories selected, the note might read:
> *Child seen for 60 minutes in day setting to work on functional use of Ⓛ UE and feeding skills. Child wore a soft spica thumb splint throughout the treatment session.*
> ***Reach/grasp/release:***
> *With min Ⓐ for facilitation of movement of elbow, child demonstrated ability to use Ⓛ UE to reach, grasp, and release 5 objects with 1–2 verbal cues per object and restriction of Ⓡ UE movement.*
> ***Feeding:***
> *Child was able to feed self Ⓘ with ~50% spillage, but demonstrated significant limitations in chewing action with ~3 rotary chews and swallowing ~90% of the food without chewing.*
> ***Attention:*** *Child required verbal cues throughout the session to maintain attention to task.*

Worksheet 6-2: Being More Concise

Revise the following note to be complete but more concise:

O: Pt. seen bedside. Client ambulated ~36 inches to shower with SBA for safety. Client instructed to complete shower while sitting. Client performed shower with SBA to manage IV line. Client able to wash upper and lower body ① and dry entire body after completing shower. Client required ~20 minutes to complete shower. Client then ambulated ~36 inches to chair and sat. Client needed verbal cues to remain seated while donning underwear and pants. Client able to dress UE ① and lower body p̄ verbal cues for sitting. Client demonstrated good sitting balance, but needed SBA for standing balance. Following shower, client stated he would like to take a nap and was assisted back into bed.

Client seen in room for skilled instruction in self-care activities. Ambulated ~3 ft. to and from shower c̄ SBA to manage IV line while ambulating and showering. Shower took ~20 minutes. Client showered and dressed c̄ verbal cues to sit. Client demonstrated good sitting balance but required SBA for balance while standing. Following shower, client assisted back into bed.

-or-

Client seen in room for skilled instruction in safe showering and dressing. Client ambulated ~3′ SBA for balance. After verbal cues to sit, client showered in 20 min c̄ SBA to manage IV lines. Dressed UE ① while seated and LE c̄ verbal cues to remain seated.

Worksheet 6-3: Being Specific About Assist Levels

Without having seen the treatment session, it is impossible to know what part of the tasks required assistance. Here are some suggestions for how the statement might have been worded:

1. Client supine → sit with min Ⓐ; bed → w/c with mod Ⓐ.
Client supine → sit with min Ⓐ to initiate activity; bed → w/c with mod Ⓐ for balance.
Client supine → sit with min Ⓐ to pull up using trapeze; bed → w/c with mod Ⓐ to lift body weight.
Client supine → sit with min Ⓐ to sequence movement; bed → w/c with mod Ⓐ to bring body to 45°.
Client supine → sit with min Ⓐ swinging legs to EOB; bed → w/c with mod Ⓐ for postural control.

2. Client required SBA in transferring w/c ↔ toilet.
Client required SBA for proper hand placement in transferring w/c ↔ toilet.
Client required SBA to remind him of steps of the transfer when transferring w/c ↔ toilet.

3. Client retrieved garments from low drawers with min Ⓐ.
Client retrieved garments from low drawers with min Ⓐ to open drawers.
Client retrieved garments from low drawers with min Ⓐ to release trigger on reacher.
Client retrieved garments from low drawers with min Ⓐ to judge halo placement in space.
Client retrieved garments from low drawers with min Ⓐ to grasp handles of drawers.

4. Brushing hair required max Ⓐ.
Brushing hair required max Ⓐ to reach back of head.
Brushing hair required max Ⓐ to flex shoulder past 35°.

5. Client completed dressing, toileting, and hygiene with min Ⓐ.
Client completed dressing, toileting, and hygiene with min Ⓐ to reach feet.
Client completed dressing, toileting, and hygiene with min Ⓐ for activities requiring fine motor dexterity.
Client completed dressing, toileting, and hygiene with min Ⓐ to adhere to hip precautions.

Worksheet 6-4: Deemphasizing the Treatment Media

1. Client played catch using bilateral UEs to facilitate grasp and release pattern.
Client worked on functional grasp/release patterns needed to manipulate household objects.

2. Resident put dirt into pot to halfway point, added seedling, and filled remainder of pot with dirt transferred by cup. Resident completed 3 more pots while standing 8 minutes before requiring a 5-minute rest. Resident resumed standing position to water completed pots for approximately 5 minutes.
Resident demonstrated standing tolerance of 13 minutes with a 5-minute break after 8 minutes in order to increase standing balance needed for ADL tasks.

3. Client painted some sungazers in crafts group to be able to see that she could do something successfully.
Client completed a series of quick-success projects to increase self-esteem.

Chapter 7

Worksheet 7-1: Justifying Continued Treatment

Which of the following require the skill of an occupational therapist?

Yes	*Evaluation of a client.*
No	*The practice of coordination and self-care skills on a daily basis.*
Yes	*Establishing measurable, behavioral, objective, and individualized goals.*
Yes	*Developing intervention plans designed to meet established goals.*
Yes	*Analyzing and modifying functional tasks/activities through the provision of adaptive equipment, or techniques.*
Yes	*Determining that the modified task is safe and effective.*
No	*Carrying out a maintenance program.*
Yes	*Teaching the client to use the breathing techniques he has learned while performing his ADL activities.*
Yes	*Providing individualized instruction to the client, family, or caregiver.*
Yes	*Modifying the intervention plan based on a reevaluation.*
Yes	*Reevaluating a client's status.*
Yes	*Providing specialized instruction to eliminate limitations in a functional activity.*
Yes	*Developing a home program and instructing caregivers.*
Yes	*Making changes in the environment.*
Yes	*Teaching compensatory skills.*
No	*Gait training.*
Yes	*Intervening with clients to eliminate safety hazards.*
No	*Presenting information handouts (such as energy conservation) without having the client perform the activity.*
No	*Routine exercise and strengthening programs.*
Yes	*Adding instruction in lower body dressing techniques to a current ADL program.*
Yes	*Teaching adaptive techniques such as one-handed shoe tying.*
Yes	*Preparing a problem list that identifies present status and potential capabilities.*

Mini-Worksheet 7-2

Problems:
> *Safety of transferring to and from the toilet.*
> *Client factors that were not WFL.*

Progress/Potential:
> *Verbalized an understanding of safety instructions.*
> *PROM ⓡ shoulder adduction WNL.*

Worksheet 7-3: Assessing Factors Not WFL

Client demonstrated difficulty with laundry and cooking tasks due to memory and sequencing deficits.
> *Memory and sequencing deficits cause difficulty c̄ home management tasks.*

Decreased level of arousal noted during morning dressing activities, requiring redirection to task.
> *↓ level of arousal limits client's ability to complete basic ADL tasks.*

Client unable to follow hip precautions during morning dressing due to memory deficits.
> *Memory deficits interfere c̄ client's ability to incorporate hip precautions into basic self-care tasks.*
> *-or-*
> *Memory deficits limit Pt.'s ability to follow hip precautions while dressing.*

Client problem-solved poorly while performing lower body dressing as evidenced by multiple attempts to button pants and don socks.
> *Client's ↓ ability to problem-solve limits her ability to dress herself s̄ Ⓐ and raises safety concerns in all ADL areas.*

Worksheet 7-4: Ellie's Development

A: Infant's inability to sit, roll, head right or push up to prone Ⓘ limits ability to engage in age-appropriate play skills and developmental exploration. Infant's decreased activity tolerance also limits her ability to engage in developmental play activities. Infant shows progress through ability to maintain facilitated positions and decrease in oxygen need. Visual tracking and scanning by turning head indicates visual awareness and orientation and show good potential for increased interaction with environment. Infant would benefit from continued facilitation of functional mobility as well as increasing strength and endurance through activities that stimulate normal development.
-or-
A: Need for facilitation and force of direction techniques limit infant's ability to perform early mobility skills. Limited mobility combined with her tolerance for less than 20 minutes of activity and the need for frequent rest breaks limit her ability to explore her environment and reach developmental milestones at a typical age. Ability to perform mobility skills with facilitation techniques, orientation to black and white design and ability to track in horizontal plane show good potential for developmental gains. Infant would benefit from continued occupational therapy services to stimulate developmental skills and from parent education in a home program.

Worksheet 7-5: Ms. D.'s Social Skills

What problems do you see in the above "S" and "O"?
Unkempt appearance
Interrupts others when talking
Does not stay on topic of conversation

What areas of occupation do these problems impact?
Social participation

What evidence of progress and/or potential do you see?
Engages in conversation
States that she understands the purpose of the group
Willingness to participate in-group
Spontaneously shared her ideas and experiences

A: *Client's unkempt appearance, interrupting behaviors, and need for redirection to topic of conversation interfere with her ability to engage in social participation with peers. Her expressed interest in groups, her willingness to engage in conversation and share her ideas show good potential to develop relationships and to express herself verbally in place of acting out. Client would benefit from participating in groups where conversational skills are stressed, from further facilitation of attention to social cues, and from assistance with ADL activities stressing hygiene and appearance.*

Chapter 8

Mini-Worksheet 8-1

P: *Continue to treat client 5x wk. for 1 week to work on safe transfers and toileting. Home program for AROM and strengthening exercises for Ⓡ shoulder will be taught. Client will demonstrate ability to transfer to toilet safely with CGA and use of walker and grab bars by the end of 5 tx. sessions.*

Worksheet 8-2: Completing the Plan for Baby Ellie

P: *Infant to be seen 3x per week for 30 minutes each visit for 3 months for stimulation of normal developmental sequences, facilitation of appropriate movement patterns, and design and modification of a home program. In order to engage in developmental play activities, infant will engage in prone play supported on elbows for 5 minutes within 3 months.*
-or-
P: *Child will be seen in the home 3 times per week to do activities that encourage postural support needed for play and environmental exploration, and for parent education in facilitating infant's development. In 1 month, child will be able to sit for 5 minutes while playing with a toy with minimal physical assist at the waist.*

Worksheet 8-3: Completing the Plan for Ms. D.

P: *Client to be seen daily for the next week to ↑ skills needed for social participation in a variety of contexts. Within 1 week, Ms. D. will demonstrate ability to engage in a 20-minute conversation without interrupting.*

-or-

P: *Client to continue social skills group 3x wk and to be given individual feedback daily on her attention to appearance and social cues. By anticipated discharge in 1 week, client will maintain neat appearance and avoid interrupting others in 3/3 1-hour group sessions.*

Chapter 9

Worksheet 9-1: Choosing Intervention Strategies

STG:

Client will be able to manage his financial affairs ① *in order to live alone after discharge. Possible intervention strategies:*
1. *Teach basic math skills (add, subtract, multiply, divide).*
2. *Role play to make change correctly.*
3. *Set up task for writing checks to pay fabricated bills.*
4. *Teach comparison shopping using a catalog.*
5. *Set up task of writing out a budget.*
6. *Set up task of balancing checkbook.*
7. *Set up experience for deciding whether a given amount of money will be enough for living expenses once a set of fabricated bills has been paid.*

Worksheet 9-2: The Case of Ginny H.

A: *Self-care deficits noted in dressing and grooming 2° to ↓ activity tolerance and standing balance, weakness in* ⑧ *shoulder flexion/abduction and ↓ problem-solving skills. ↓ standing balance impairs ability to transfer and ambulate* ① *and safely. Weakness noted in* ⓡ *grasp and lateral/tripod pinch and ↓ coordination affecting fine motor coordination tasks. These problem areas negatively impact client's ability to be* ① *and safe in ADL tasks. Rehab potential is good for returning home with caregiver assistance. Client would benefit from treatment to increase activity tolerance, dynamic standing balance, and safety for ADL tasks.*

P: *Pt. to be seen b.i.d. for 45 min for 3 wks. to ↑* ① *in self-care activities through instruction and use of adaptive equipment/techniques, to ↑ activity tolerance, standing balance and* ① *in transfers for functional mobility and to ↑* ⓡ *hand strength in order to be able to dress and toilet self* ①. *By end of 1 wk. client will be able to transfer safely and* ① *bed to bedside commode and manage clothing with SBA at walker s̄ losing balance.*

LTG: **In 3 wks. client will be:**
1. ① *in dressing and grooming.*
2. ① *and safe in toileting using walker and bedside commode.*

STG: **In 1 wk. client will:**
1. *Demonstrate ability to don/doff gown and robe with min* ⓐ *for set-up and verbal cues.*
2. *↑ ADL tolerance as demonstrated by ability to tolerate >10 min of activity first while sitting, then standing with one 30-sec. rest break.*
3. *Transfer safely → bedside commode with SBA to manage clothing with no more than 2 verbal cues.*
4. **In 2 wks. client will** *be assessed for possible home visit and home equipment needs.*

Signature: Gayla G., OTR/L

Treatment Plan
Name: *Ginny H.*   **Age:** *87*   **Sex:** *F*   **Physician:** *B. Garrett, MD*
Onset: *4/22/05*   **Date of Referral:** *5/2/05*   **Date of Initial Evaluation:** *5/3/05*
Diagnosis: Ⓛ *subdural hematoma on 4/22/05, hx. of HBP, hearing loss*
Referral Source: *Nursing*
Frequency and Duration of Treatment: *b.i.d. x3 wks.*
Strengths: Ⓘ *in self-care prior to CVA; able to ambulate c̄ walker, intact sensation except for* Ⓡ *hand stereognosis; all UE AROM WNL or WFL.*
Functional Problems:

1.   ↓ *ability to perform self-care tasks due to impaired problem solving, ↓ coordination,*
     ↓ *stereognosis, ↓ standing balance.*
2.   *Safety concerns due to fatigue during ADL tasks and ↓ dynamic balance during clothing management and transfers when toileting.*

Frequency and Duration of Treatment: *b.i.d. x3 wks.*

Long-Term Goals	Short-Term Goals	Interventions
By anticipated discharge (5/22/05) client will be Ⓘ in dressing and grooming.	By 5/10/05 client will: 1. Demonstrate ability to don/doff gown and robe with min Ⓐ for set-up and verbal cues. 2. ↑ ADL tolerance as demonstrated by ability to tolerate >10 min of activity while sitting or standing with one 30-sec. rest break.	Instruct client on upper body dressing techniques and have client demonstrate over-the-head and button-up methods, first in sitting and progress to standing. Provide tactile cues to use alternative techniques. Have client problem solve for next step of dressing or grooming tasks in sequence using visual and then verbal cues as needed. Ask client what to do next or why this is not working now. Engage client in reaching activities that provide a graded challenge to balance. Engage client in activities that ↑ AROM and fine-motor tasks such as buttoning and zipping that are graded for level of difficulty in coordination. Educate client on identifying signs of fatigue. Plan rest breaks as needed to ↓ fatigue. Perform tabletop activities including self-care tasks with time increasing as tolerated. Perform deep breathing exercises and instruct in energy conservation techniques.

By anticipated discharge (5/22/05) client will be ① and safe in toileting using adaptive equipment (walker and 3-in-1 commode).	*3. Client will transfer safely ↔ 3-in-1 commode when toileting with SBA to manage clothing and no more than 2 verbal cues in 1 week.* *4. Client will be assessed for possible home visit and home equipment needs in 2 weeks.*	*Instruct client in safe transfer techniques; reinforce compliance when transferring ↔ bed, armchairs, 3-in-1 commode, and mat for therapeutic activities, strengthen exercises, toileting or dressing activities.* *Provide ® UE strengthening and AROM through reaching and wt. bearing activities such as: reaching at sink for grooming and dressing items in graded challenging positions; pushing up from armchair and bedside commode; and table top activities of interest that require alternating support on one arm while actively reaching with the other.* *Interview client and daughter regarding home environment; explore and discuss equipment use & placement in home; discuss support services needed if discharge to home is warranted. Schedule a home visit for assessment of client's ability to manage in home environment.*

Discharge Plan: *To home if environmental adaptations and support of caregiver and/or services are available. If client is not① in self-care activities by 5/22/05, the recommendation would be to discharge to an assisted living facility for 2 to 3 wks. until self-care goals are met.*

Signature: Gayla G., OTR/L

Worksheet 9-3: Planning Interventions for Sarah

Problem #1: Exacerbation of depression including low self-esteem and a recent suicide attempt leading to safety concerns in an independent living situation.

LTG #1: By anticipated discharge in 4 days, Sarah will demonstrate an increase in self-esteem by a neat appearance, making eye contact during conversation at least once daily, and verbally identifying a positive resource or coping strategy she has used successfully in the past.

Goals Group

Listen attentively to what Sarah is saying when she shares her goal.
Offer eye contact and offer Sarah the opportunity to make eye contact in return before cueing her.
Help Sarah identify the relationship between her values and her daily goals (i.e., a goal to wash her hair is related to valuing a neat clean appearance).
Help Sarah break down larger goals (such as "be happy") into smaller accomplishable increments.
Show respect for Sarah's choices.
Provide feedback on Sarah's successes in meeting her daily goals.
Facilitate goal choices that show increased self-esteem.
Compliment Sarah on her appearance when any part of her appearance shows more attention to her self-care.
Facilitate goal choices that involve taking care of herself.

Stress Management Group

Welcome Sarah by greeting her warmly, sitting by her, or smiling.
Offer opportunities to find value in herself through visualization and imagery.
Help Sarah identify stresses that led to her recent suicide attempt.

Help Sarah identify both successful and unsuccessful stress relief strategies she has used in the past.
Brainstorm ways of handling stressful situations that seem overwhelming before those situations become life-threatening.
Use positive affirmations.
Provide practice for a variety of stress management strategies.

IADL Group

Identify positives about each person through:
> *Group discussion*
> *Art activities (draw your best quality, collage, etc.)*
> *Games*
Use a peer feedback activity that identifies qualities peers appreciate in each other.
Offer quick success projects, such as putting together jewelry, making bookmarks, or completing small kits.
Ask Sarah for her ideas about how to best use the group time.
Note aspects of Sarah's work that are executed with competence.
In a group that is all women, learn to apply makeup or style hair.

Problem #2: Stress related to recent role changes result in Sarah's inability to focus her thoughts sufficiently to make decisions for her daily life.

LTG #2: Sarah will have a plan in place for making decisions regarding her two most important current life decisions by discharge in 4 days.

Goals Group

Identify a small accomplishable goal for the day.
Help Sarah identify what is realistic to accomplish in 1 day.
Write that goal on a card for Sarah to carry with her throughout the day.
Make a verbal contract with Sarah to accomplish her goal.
Teach the relationship between setting daily goals and making larger life decisions.
Follow up daily on Sarah's goal for the day.
Encourage Sarah to make goals related to her major life stressors.

Stress Management Group

Help Sarah identify triggers in her environment that cause a stress reaction.
Use cognitive reframing.
Help Sarah bring her thoughts to the present moment and to come back to the present moment when she drifts into the past and future.
Use movement, such as stretching or progressive relaxation, to help Sarah focus on the task at hand.

IADL Group

Ask Sarah about strategies she uses to focus her mind.
Plan group topics around Sarah's current issues, such as:
> *Ways of getting to sleep*
> *Overcoming loneliness*
> *Feeling worthwhile*
Use a cognitively stimulating activity to help Sarah focus.
Brainstorm strategies for making good decisions and rank these in effectiveness.
Ask Sarah to identify one major decision needing to be made, and list pluses and minuses of each possible course of action.
Role play a decision-making situation.
Use games that require decision making.
Adapt tasks so that Sarah will be able to concentrate on a task long enough to complete it.

Problem #3: Sarah does not recognize anger building and does not have useful ways of expressing it, resulting in expressions of anger that damage self, relationships, and property.

LTG #3: By anticipated discharge in 4 days, Sarah will identify feelings, behaviors, and bodily sensations that are associated with varying stages of anger.

Goals Group

Use active listening to help Sarah identify feelings related to her goals.
Ask Sarah about daily incidents involving anger and encourage goals for useful solutions if incidents arise.

Stress Management Group

Use stress management techniques that focus on body sensations.
Teach Sarah to focus on the breath to bring her to the present moment, to relax, and to enhance sleep.
Invite Sarah to identify and express feelings that arise during the exercises.
Use sounds and recordings that activate the parasympathetic nervous system.
Identify strategies for restful sleep and encourage her to practice these at night.

IADL Group

Teach anger management strategies.
Help Sarah identify feelings that arise during the group.
Use sounds and language to elicit feelings.
Use art activities to explore and express feelings.
Identify stressors that trigger anger through:
> *Group discussion*
> *Adapted games*
> *Art*

Role play situations around anger and frustration.
Identify social supports (friends, family, support groups, crisis lines) to use when angry.
Teach the use of lightheartedness and humor to dissipate anger.
Teach and role play problem solving.
Coach Sarah as she practices managing anger with phone calls and visitors.
Use listening dyads.
Teach the use of an "anger continuum" to recognize varying degrees and experiences of anger.

Chapter 10

Worksheet 10-1: Initial Evaluation Report

Background Data

Criteria	Compliance
Are all of the following present: name, date of birth, gender? What are the applicable diagnoses?	Age is given in place of DOB. CVA; r/o OBS.
Who referred the client to OT, on what date, what services requested?	Dr. Grantham referred her for evaluation and treatment. No referral date is given.
What is the funding source?	Not noted, but she is 68 which implies Medicare.
What length of stay is anticipated?	2 weeks.

Why is the client seeking occupational therapy services?	She wants to go home.
Are there any secondary problems, pre-existing conditions, contraindications, or precautions that will impact therapy?	Diabetes.

Occupational History and Profile

Is there an occupational history/profile? Is it adequate?	There is a brief occupational profile. More information can be obtained during tx.
Which areas of occupation are currently successful and which are problematic?	No successful areas noted. ADL and IADL tasks are problematic.
What factors hinder her performance in areas of occupation? What factors support her performance in areas of occupation?	Hinder: ↓ problem solving ability, slow cognitive responses ↓ ability to initiate and sequence tasks. Some client factors not WNL. Support: A nearby daughter who is willing to visit daily and assist with transportation, intact sensation, motor planning and perception WFL, able to stand and transfer with CGA, 1-story home, sedentary hobbies, motivation to go home.
What are the client's priorities?	To go back to her own home.
What areas of occupation will be targeted for intervention? Do these match the client's priorities?	ADL and IADL, which do match the client's priorities.
What are the targeted outcomes?	Discharge to home. Modified Ⓘ and safety in ADL activities.

Results of the Assessment

What types of assessments were used?	Mini-mental status, ADL evaluation, manual muscle test, sensation, observation, interview, AROM.
What were the results of the assessments?	Results are clearly noted on the evaluation form and in the "A".
What client factors, contextual aspects, and activity demands are identified as needing attention?	Client factors: ↓ AROM and strength in the Ⓛ UE, ↓ activity tolerance, ↓ problem solving, sequencing, and memory. Context: Lives alone and daughter unable to provide supervision; needs cues for orientation. Activity demands: Needs cues to initiate and sequence activities and to problem solve.
What factors (strengths, supports) facilitate her occupational performance?	Supportive daughter.
How confident is this OT that her evaluation results are valid?	Confidence level not noted.
Is OT appropriate for this client?	Yes.

Worksheet 10-2: Intervention Plan

Criteria	Compliance
Is client information present on the evaluation or intervention plan (name, age, gender, precautions, contraindications)?	No precautions or contraindications are noted; client is diabetic. Client info noted on evaluation form.
Are the types of interventions to be used identified?	Yes.
Are the intervention goals and objectives measurable?	Yes.
Are the goals and objectives directly related to the client's ability to engage in the desired occupations?	Yes.
What is the anticipated frequency/duration of services?	45-minute sessions 5x wk. for 2 weeks.
What is the discontinuation criteria?	Ability to live at home safely without supervision.
What is the anticipated discharge location?	Home.
What is the anticipated plan for follow-up care?	Not noted.
What is the name and position of the person overseeing the plan of care?	Not noted.
What date was the plan developed, and what date(s) was it modified or reviewed?	Developed 2/3/05 Not yet modified or reviewed.

Worksheet 10-3: Treatment, Visit, or Contact Notes

Criteria	Compliance
Is client information (name, date of birth, gender, diagnosis, precautions, and/or contraindications) present?	No date of birth or diagnosis given. In an acute care setting the client information is commonly stamped onto each page of the health record with an addressograph card. No precautions or contraindications given.
What is the date and time of the contact?	4/14/05 at 8:30 AM.
What type of contact is this?	Client contact for ADL interventions.
What are the names and positions of the persons involved in the contact?	John B., client Bonnie B., OTR/L
Is there a summary of the intervention or the information communicated during the contact?	Yes.
Is the client's participation in the contact (or the reason service was missed) present?	Yes.

Is there an indication of the environmental or task modification, assistive or adaptive devices used or fabricated, training, education, or consultation provided, and persons present?	No adaptations in this intervention.

Worksheet 10-4: Progress Notes

Criteria	Compliance
Is client information (name, date of birth, gender, diagnosis, precautions, and/or contraindications) present?	No. Since this is an inpatient health record, this information would not necessarily be written by the therapist onto each progress note sheet.
What is the frequency of services? How long have services been provided?	8 groups per week offered; client attended 6/8. The note covers one week. SOC not noted.
What techniques and strategies were used? What programs or training were provided to the client or caregiver?	Assertion group; communication group; IADL group. No training to caregivers as yet; client to talk to husband about leisure plans.
Were any environmental or task modifications provided? Any adaptive equipment or orthotic devices?	Client needs structure.
What other pertinent client updates are given?	Leisure plan to be developed and discussed with husband and social worker; goals updated.
What is the client's response to occupational therapy services?	Shares without prompting; spontaneously answered a question; offered to help a peer; increased attention to appearance; unprompted attendance.
What is the client's progress toward his goals?	Two goals met, one goal continued, one goal discontinued. Progress as noted above.
What areas of occupation are being addressed?	Social participation, IADL, self-care, leisure.
What recommendations are made and why? What is the client's input to the intervention plan?	Plan structured day to prevent relapse; attend groups 2 more days. Leisure plan recommended; no notation of client's input to changes.

Worksheet 10-5: Reevaluation Reports

Criteria	Compliance
Is client information (name, date of birth, gender, diagnosis, precautions, and or contraindications) present?	Everything present; no contraindications or precautions noted.
What is the updated status of current areas of occupation that are successful or problematic?	Able to do more ADL, IADL, and work tasks successfully. Still has difficulty with locked doors; some client factors still not WNL.
What contexts support occupations? What contexts hinder occupations?	Ergonomic keyboard at work. Lives alone and does not have help with areas that are still problematic.

Is there a summary of any new health/work/educational information?	Client education and strengthening. Obtained ergonomically shaped keyboard.
What are the updates/changes to the client's priorities and targeted outcomes?	No changes in client priorities.
What was the focus (purpose) of the re-evaluation?	Determination of continued need for occupational therapy services.
What assessments were used?	Goniometry; grip strength; interview, visual inspection for edema.
How do the results compare with the previous evaluation results?	Improvement in client factors, ADLs, IADLs, and work status. Decrease in pain.
What is the client's response to the re-evaluation?	No reported response to reevaluation.
Is there an interpretation of the summary and comparison of results with previous evaluation results?	Yes.
What changes to occupational therapy services, goals, or referrals will be made as a result of the reevaluation?	Services will be discontinued.

Worksheet 10-6: Transition Plan

Criteria	Compliance
Is client information (name, date of birth, gender diagnosis, precautions, and/or contraindications present?	Yes.
What is the client's current performance in occupations?	At a 4-month level, working on reach, grasp, and release, rolling, ability to sustain anti-gravity positions. Visual regard, midline orientation, and visually directed reach.
What is the current setting?	Birth-to-Three program.
What is the setting into which the client is transferring?	Preschool program.
What is the reason for the transition?	Age.
What is the time frame in which the transition will occur?	May (1 month).
What activities are to be carried out during the transition plan?	Home program.
What recommendations are made for occupational therapy services in the new setting?	Reevaluate; continue OT, PT, and speech therapy.
What is the rationale for this recommendation?	To stimulate her progress through the developmental sequence.
What modifications, accommodations, assistive technology, or environmental modifications are needed?	None noted.

Worksheet 10-7: Discharge Summary

Criteria	Compliance
Is client information (name, date of birth, gender diagnosis, precautions, and/or contraindications) present?	No.
What was the date of initial service? What was the date of end of service?	1/25/05 2/19/05
What was the client's progress toward goals?	↑ in independence. Met all treatment goals.
What was the client's beginning and ending status regarding ability to engage in occupations?	Beginning: Mod (A) for ADL task except for max (A) in bathing. Ending SBA for all ADL tasks, except (I) in toileting.
What is the client's assessment of occupational therapy services?	Pleased (in SOAP format). Not given in facility format.
What are the recommendations pertaining to the consumer's future needs?	Continue HEP. Outpatient physical therapy. Two pieces of adaptive equipment and home modifications recommended.

Chapter 12

Mini-Worksheet 12-1: Writing Problem Statements

Pt. unable to dress LE (I) due to trunk instability.
    Tell what assist level is needed rather than saying unable to dress (I).
    Say "lower body" rather than LE, since the client is dressing more than just the extremity.
    If there is one particular part of the task that requires assistance, specify that. For example:
    Client needs mod (A) to maintain balance while dressing lower body due to trunk instability.

Child doesn't tolerate very much classroom activity due to ↓ activity tolerance.
    Specify how much "very much" is.
    Tell what kind of classroom activity. For example:
    Child tolerates less than ½ hour of desk work in the classroom due to ↓ activity tolerance.

Consumer acts out.
    Specify what is meant by "acting out".
    Specify what area of occupation is problematic because of the acting out.
    Specify the underlying factor that is responsible for the acting out. For example:
    Consumer cuts or burns extremities when upset, resulting in frequent emergency room visits and difficulty resolving conflict with spouse.
    -or-
    Consumer has difficulty sustaining friendships due to inappropriate verbal and physical actions.

Worksheet 12-2: Writing Functional and Measurable Goals

Client will pivot while standing with SBA during toilet transfers in 1 day.

> *Reword this goal for clarity. For example:*
> *Client will be able to perform standing pivot transfer to toilet SBA for safety within 1 day.*
> *-or-*
> *Client will be able to go w/c → toilet standing pivot SBA within 1 day.*

Client will be min Ⓐ in dressing, UE and LE, in 10 days.

> *This goal needs to be written in terms of what the client needs, rather than stating that he will be a particular assist level. It is a small item that shows more respect to word the goal statement so that it acknowledges that the client is more than his ability to dress himself. Specify the conditions under which the client will dress himself (including what parts of the task need assistance), rather than that he will dress only his upper and lower extremities. For example:*
> *Client will be able to dress self sitting EOB with min Ⓐ to pull pants over hips within 10 days.*

Deemphasizing the Treatment Media.

> Client will place 8 half-inch screws and washers on a block of wood with holes by next treatment session.
> *By the end of 2nd treatment session, client will demonstrate ability to handle small objects needed to return to work by placing 8 half-inch screws into a block of wood in <5 minutes.*

> Client will make a clock using the appropriate materials by anticipated discharge in 1 week.
> *Pt. will demonstrate the ability to grasp/place release objects of various sized needed for IADL activities by assembling a clock Ⓘ by anticipated discharge in 2 weeks.*
> *-or-*
> *Client will demonstrate ability to follow written directions for IADL tasks by assembling a clock from written instructions within 1 week.*

> Client will stay in his chair without reminders and spend at least 30 minutes lacing the leather billfold during the 45-minute craft group session in 2 weeks.
> *Within 1 month, client will demonstrate attention to task needed to qualify for sheltered workshop program by staying in his chair without reminders and attending to craft project for 30 minutes or more.*

Worksheet 12-3: SOAPing Your Note

O	*Client supine → sit in bed Ⓘ.*
O	*Client moved kitchen items from counter to cabinet Ⓘ using Ⓛ hand.*
A	*Problems include decreased coordination, strength, sensation, and proprioception in left hand which create safety risks in home management tasks.*
S	*Client reports that his fingers are stiff this morning and that he is having trouble handling small items like buttons.*
A	*Client's ↑ of 15 minutes in activity tolerance for UE activities permits her to prepare a light meal Ⓘ.*
O	*Child seen in OT clinic for 1-hour evaluation of hand function.*
P	*In order to return to work, client will demonstrate an increase of 10# grasp in Ⓛ hand by 1/3/05.*
A	*Decreased proprioception and motor planning limit client's ability to dress upper body.*
P	*Continue retrograde massage to Ⓡ hand for edema control.*
A	*Client's correct identification of inappropriate positioning 100% of the time would indicate memory WFL.*

S   *Client reports that she cannot remember hip precautions.*
A   *Client would benefit from further instruction to incorporate total hip precautions into lower body dressing, bathing, and hygiene.*
A   *Learning was evident by client's ability to improve with repetition.*
O   *Client does not make eye contact during group session.*
A   *Client's request to take rest breaks demonstrates knowledge of her limitations in endurance.*
O   *Client wrote bank check for correct amount to pay electric bill with two verbal cues.*
A   *3+ muscle grade of extension in Ⓡ wrist extensors this week shows good progress toward goals.*
O   *Client completed weight shifts of trunk x10 in each of anterior, posterior, left, and right lateral directions in preparation for standing to perform home management tasks.*
A   *Unkempt appearance in mock interview situation indicates poor judgment and self-concept.*

Worksheet 12-4: Writing the "S"—Subjective

Client reports arthritis in Ⓡ shoulder and knee, pain on weight bearing. During transfer, client requested specific adjustments such as sliding board placement, proximity to bed, and approaching bed from the affected side. Fatigue reported after transfer.
-or-
Pt. reports significant arthritis in shoulder and knee, and prefers to approach transfers from the affected side. Pt. reports "It hurts to stand on my leg." Pt. also stated w/c → bed sliding board are the most difficult, and reported fatigue after transfer.
-or-
Client reports arthritis is Ⓡ shoulder and knee and pain bearing weight on Ⓡ LE. Pt. able to verbalize needs regarding transfer (placement of board and approach from affected side). Client reports fatigue after transfer.

Worksheet 12-5: Writing Good Opening Lines

Client seen in room for 45 minutes for morning self-care activities.
Client seen in room for 45 minutes to increase Ⓘ in ADL activities, to decrease safety concerns during functional mobility, and to provide instruction on proper use of adaptive equipment.
-or-
Client seen in hospital room for 45 minutes for education on use of adaptive equipment and toilet transfers during morning self-care activities.
-or-
Client seen beside for 45 minutes for education on safety concerns during ADLs and skilled instruction in use of adaptive equipment.
-or-
Client seen bedside for 45 minutes for skilled instruction in use of adaptive equipment and hip precaution education during performance of morning ADLs and transfers to and from toilet.

Client seen at workshop for 1 hr. to work on job skills.
Client seen at workshop for 1 hr. to address cognitive, sensory, and bilateral integration barriers to performing work tasks effectively.
-or-
Client seen at workshop for 1 hr. to work on sequencing, bilateral coordination, concentration and sensory awareness while completing work task of package handling.
-or-
Client seen at workshop for 1 hr. to improve sequencing skills, increase bilateral coordination, and decrease distractibility at work.

-or-

Client seen @ workshop for 1 hr. for skilled instruction in task sequencing, bilateral coordination, and techniques to decrease sensory registration to increase attention for job skills.

Client seen bedside for 30 minutes for morning dressing.

Client seen bedside for 30 minutes for morning dressing to improve balance, bilateral motor control, functional mobility, and safety in order to return home.

-or-

Client seen bedside for 30 minutes to increase balance and Ⓑ motor control for safety during basic ADLs and use of manual wheelchair.

-or-

Client seen bedside for 30 minutes to increase balance and bilateral control of upper extremities during dressing and functional mobility.

-or-

Client seen at bedside for 30 minutes to enhance balance and Ⓑ motor tasks involving UE to increase safety during dressing and w/c mobility.

Client seen in kitchen for 1 hr. to work on Ⓘ in cooking.

Client seen in kitchen for 1 hr. to increase dynamic standing balance and increase awareness of affected UE for safety in cooking.

-or-

Client seen in kitchen for 1 hr. to address safety concerns regarding balance and Ⓛ UE neglect.

-or-

Client seen in kitchen for 1 hr. to increase standing balance and attention affected UE to increase safety while cooking.

-or-

Client seen in kitchen for 1 hr. to work on cooking tasks with attention to standing balance, affected UE position, and safety.

-or-

Client seen in kitchen for 1 hr. for skilled instruction in kitchen safety to improve standing balance and attention to affected UE.

Mini-Worksheet 12-6

No   *Client required max Ⓐ x2 bed → bedside commode and bed → w/c and was dependent for pericare.*

Yes   *Child required HOH Ⓐ to stay in the lines when following path with crayon.*

Yes   *Client needed mod verbal cues to participate in discussion in life skills group.*

No   *Resident min Ⓐ to don sock due to pain.*

Worksheet 12-7: Writing the "O"—Objective

First, an opening line is needed stating where, for how long, and for what purpose the client was seen. One possibility is:

> *Client seen in room for skilled instruction in ADL tasks and assessment of splinting needs.*
> -or-
> *Client seen bedside for skilled instruction in compensatory dressing techniques and evaluation of splinting needs.*

Second, the categories could be reduced to three—toileting, dressing, and splinting evaluation.

Third, it would be helpful to know what part of the task needed assistance.

Fourth, the UE and LE wording is not inclusive enough, since the client is dressing the upper and lower body rather than just the extremities.

Finally, under hand status there is no functional component, and "index finger greatest amount" is not very informative.

Worksheet 12-8: Differentiating Between Observations and Assessments

O   *Client is unable to don AFO and shoe Ⓘ for ambulation.*
A   *Inability to don AFO and shoe Ⓘ prevent her from ambulating safely around the house to live alone.*
A   *Decreased sensory tolerance limits the client's attention to task in the classroom.*
O   *Client requires verbal cues to stay on task due to decreased sensory tolerance.*
O   *Client was unable to incorporate breathing and energy conservation techniques, requiring several verbal prompts to complete task.*
A   *Inability to incorporate breathing techniques and energy conservation techniques into basic ADL tasks s̄ verbal prompts limits her ability to live alone Ⓘ p̄ discharge.*

> *Decreased memory and sequencing abilities limit client's ability to perform IADL activities such as laundry and cooking tasks.*
> -or-
> *Memory and sequencing deficits interfere with client's ability to perform IADLs such as laundry and cooking Ⓘ, and limit her ability to return to an Ⓘ living situation.*
> -or-
> *Deficits in memory and sequencing limit the client's ability to do many IADLs, for example laundry and cooking.*
> -or-
> *Deficits in memory and sequencing leads to difficulty with IADL tasks such as laundry and cooking tasks necessary for household management.*

Client unable to complete homemaking tasks or basic self-care activities Ⓘ due to ↓ endurance and not following hip precautions.

> *Decreased endurance and inability to follow hip precautions limits client's ability to complete homemaking tasks and self-care activities Ⓘ .*
> -or-
> *Failure to follow hip precautions and decreased endurance interfere with client's ability to complete homemaking tasks and decrease ability to successfully complete basic self-care activities Ⓘ .*

-or-
Decreased endurance and failure to follow hip precautions prevent client from performing homemaking and BADL tasks Ⓘ and safely.

After the use of behavior modification techniques, client displayed courteous behavior for the remainder of the treatment session.

You could take a positive or a negative approach to this one.

Positive:

> *Client's ability to behave courteously with the aid of behavior modification techniques indicates good potential for improving problem behaviors in school.*
>
> *-or-*
>
> *Client's positive response to behavior modification techniques shows good potential to meet social participation goals.*

Negative:

> *The need for behavior modification techniques to elicit courteous behavior limit client's ability to interact appropriately with peers in social settings.*
>
> *-or-*
>
> *Client's need for instruction in behavior modification limits his ability to communicate with others effectively in social situations.*

Worksheet 12-9: Problems, Progress, and Rehab Potential

Problems:

After reading through this note, several problems stood out for this OT:

- Dynamic sitting balance
- Weight shifting
- Posture
- Transfers

(The four above are related to safety and functional mobility)

- Decreased AROM in Ⓡ UE (mod Ⓐ to reach)
- Cognition

On thinking a little further, she decided that the "cognition" problem might really be one of the following, since he does seem to understand the goal of the activity.

- Short-term memory
- Motor planning
- Problem solving
- Initiation

Finally the OT decides that the problem with initiation is probably some combination of problem solving and motor planning deficit.

Progress/Rehab Potential/Strengths

- Ability to understand the treatment goal

The therapist then groups the problems according to the impact they have on the client's occupational performance. She decides that the first three cause difficulty with functional mobility, and are of particular concern because they create safety issues. The motor planning and initiation problem is a concern in the area of self-care, as is the problem with decrease in AROM of the right UE. The need for continual instruction, whether it is a problem with short-term memory or with his ability to problem solve, is likely to require a lot of attention from a caregiver at home. The client does, however, understand why he is doing the task she has given him, as long as the goals are not set too high, he should be able to make good progress in rehabilitation. Her assessment and plan read as follows:

A: Deficits in postural control, dynamic sitting balance, and weight shifting raise safety concerns when transferring. ↓ AROM and motor planning ability negatively impact ability to perform self-care tasks. A need for continual instruction to prevent unsafe performance of ADL tasks requires a high level of caregiver assistance. Client's ability to understand treatment goal indicates good rehab potential for the goals established. Client would benefit from continued skilled instruction in activities to ↑ balance, safe functional mobility, and Ⓘ in ADL tasks.

P: Continue tx daily for 3 weeks for skilled instruction in self care tasks and safe transfers. In 3 weeks client will be able to transfer safely from wheelchair to bed or toilet c̄ min Ⓐ for balance.

Another OT might assess the session a little differently. For example:

A: Problems include deficits in motor planning, movement initiation, cognition, and muscle weakness in Ⓡ UE which ↓ safety in ADL tasks and functional mobility. Activity tolerance has improved since yesterday from <1 minute to >3 minutes without a rest break. Client would benefit from skilled OT to increase balance, functional mobility, and grasp/release activities with involved UE in order to ↑ Ⓘ in self-care activities.

P: Continue tx. b.i.d. for ½ hour sessions to work on Ⓡ UE movement and cognitive retraining in order to complete grooming activities with min Ⓐ. Client will be able to brush teeth with min Ⓐ by the end of 5th tx. session.
-or-
A: Decreased functional use of the Ⓡ UE, decreased sitting balance, and difficulty with sequencing and problem-solving limit ability to perform ADLs. Increased shoulder flexion and motor planning since initial evaluation and increased understanding of treatment activities would indicate good rehab potential. Client would benefit from continued skilled OT to increase functional AROM, exercises in grasp, exercises in weight shifting to improve dynamic sitting balance, and evaluation of both cognitive status and ability to initiate activity in order to increase Ⓘ in ADL tasks.

P: Continue b.i.d. for 30 minute sessions for 2 weeks to increase dynamic sitting balance in preparation for ADL training. Client will be able to reach for grooming items placed slightly beyond arm's reach without losing balance 3/4 times within 2 weeks.

Worksheet 12-10: The School Note

Problems
- Visual tracking and eye convergence
- Muscle tone/upper body strength
- Bilateral coordination
- Fine motor skills
- Poor handwriting
- UE weakness
- Proximal stability

Progress/Potential
- Improvement in ability to form letters within lines
- 90% accuracy from memory of some letters
- Handwriting improvement

A: Decreased upper body strength and proximal stability limit the child's ability to use his upper extremities in an accurate and coordinated manner in class. Lack of fine motor and bilateral coordination limit the child's accuracy in schoolwork (including handwriting, art, and play activities). Inaccuracy in visual tracking and eye convergence interfere with ability to form letters and numbers or to complete written work from a book or blackboard at grade level. Lack of visual tracking and convergence skills also limits ability to perform age-appropriate games safely. Improvement in accuracy of letter formation since last note and ability to remember 6 letter shapes indicate good progress and good potential to meet IEP goals. Child would benefit from continued work on postural stability to support functional UE use, as well as from continued work on visual and motor skills needed for classroom activities.

P: Continue occupational therapy twice weekly for 30-minute sessions for the remainder of the school year. By the end of the school year child will be able to write all letters of the alphabet within line boundaries 3/3 tries.

Worksheet 12-11: Mr. S.'s Communication Skills

Problems
- Communication (changes the subject rather than answer the question)
- Assertion (does not define, and states he does not wish to use)
- Non-responsive to group role-play activity
- Sitting with head down and eyes closed during group
- Self-expression (verbal and nonverbal)

These behaviors limit his appropriate social participation and his freedom to leave the institution.

Progress/Potential
- Neat appearance
- Attended group and was on time
- Remained for duration of group

A: Poor ability to define assertive behavior and the statement that he prefers manipulation and aggression as relational skills limit Mr. S.'s ability to resolve conflicts and relate to others effectively, thus limiting his ability to function ① in a community setting. Sitting with head down and eyes closed seems to be a strong nonverbal statement of his desire to be non-participatory. His lack of participation in group activity limit his ability to use the group time to problem-solve ways of changing this relational/communication skill. Ability to manage time, willingness to remain in group until the end, and good dressing/grooming skills indicate good potential to meet stated goal of moving to the next level of least restrictive environment.

P: Client to be seen in all regularly scheduled psychosocial skills groups for 1 month, in addition to 1:1 sessions on unit to offer opportunities to relate effectively. By the end of 1 month, client will participate in at least one activity in assertion group.

Worksheet 12-12: The "Almost" Note

Here we have a note that seems good on the surface, but demonstrates some problems in critical thinking. The most outstanding problem with this note is that the OT is mixing her "O" data and her "A" data.

First, it would have helped the "S" if the therapist had asked pertinent questions, such as what her pain levels were.

Second, there is nothing in the "O" to show that skilled occupational therapy is being provided. The list of observations of assist levels fails to provide the richness of the skill used in treatment. The therapist erroneously puts some of that information in the "A" section, rather than assessing her data. In the "A" she tells us:

Client (I) in dressing while sitting EOB, but is min (A) in dressing when standing with a walker. (L) UE AROM is WFL but (R) UE has deficits noted in shoulder flexion. Client SBA in bed mobility when rolling to unaffected side and min (A) in sit → stand 2° to ↑ UE strength. Client needs SBA for transfer to unaffected side in pivot transfer bed → w/c and min (A) w/c → toilet.

Even if this information were moved into the "O", there is nothing to tell us what part of the task the assistance was for. The OT uses a nonstandard abbreviation "*VCs*". She means verbal cues, but since *VC* is a standard health term meaning *vital capacity*, it is inappropriate in its usage here.

Third, the coordination deficits mentioned in the "A" section come out of the blue. There is no mention of coordination in the opening statement *...for work on dressing and functional mobility* nor is it mentioned in the "O". Thus the statement that coordination deficits are one of the problems noted and the statement that the client would benefit from coordination exercises are unsubstantiated. Remember not to introduce any new information in the "A" section of your note.

There is no real assessment of the meaning of the data found in the "S" and the "O." There is a short list of problem areas, but no assessment of their impact of ability to engage in meaningful occupation, and no assessment of the rehab potential shown by the client's willingness to "*do whatever it takes to get out of the hospital.*"

The best thing for this therapist to do is to rewrite the "O" section, providing a more comprehensive picture of the treatment session. Then she needs to assess her data based on her observations. There needs to be an indication of how the observed data impact the occupational performance of the client, before the statements about what the client would benefit from.

Depending on the assessment she makes, the plan to work on balance may be appropriate, or it may be only one of the things to be addressed.

Index

WAIT
...There's More!

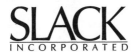